the *fourth* trimester

the *fourth* trimester

a postpartum guide
to *healing* your body,
balancing your emotions
& *restoring* your vitality

KIMBERLY ANN JOHNSON

SHAMBHALA
BOULDER
2017

Shambhala Publications, Inc.
4720 Walnut Street
Boulder, CO 80301
www.shambhala.com

9 8 7 6 5

Printed in the United States of America

⊗ This edition is printed on acid-free paper that meets the American
National Standards Institute Z39.48 Standard.
✿ Shambhala makes every effort to print on recycled paper.
For more information please visit www.shambhala.com.

Shambhala Publications is distributed worldwide by
Penguin Random House, Inc., and its subsidiaries.

Designed by Allison Meierding

Library of Congress Cataloging-in-Publication Data

Names: Johnson, Kimberly Ann.
Title: The fourth trimester: a postpartum guide to healing your body,
balancing your emotions, and restoring your vitality / Kimberly Ann Johnson.
Description: First edition. | Boulder: Shambhala, 2017. | Includes
bibliographical references and index.
Identifiers: LCCN 2017007166 | ISBN 9781611804003 (pbk.: alk. paper)
Subjects: LCSH: Mothers—Psychology. | Mothers—Life skills guides. |
Mothers—Health and hygiene. | Mother and child.
Classification: LCC HQ759 .J6437 2017 | DDC 155.6/463—dc23
LC record available at https://lccn.loc.gov/2017007166

For Cecilia, the sweetest answer to my lifelong prayer to be a mother.

For Mom, the birth would have been different with you there.

Salve Iemanja, santa da minha cabeça e moradora do meu coração.

A mother's body against a child's body make a place.
It says you are here. Without this body there is no place.

—EVE ENSLER from *In the Body of the World*

You think because you understand "one" you must
also understand "two," because one and one make two.
But you must also understand "and."

—RUMI

contents

foreword

.... ❧ ....

Get your body back after baby. Right? That's what we hear from other moms, that's what we see in the media—perfect images of stunning pregnant celebrities who, mere weeks after delivery, somehow seem to have returned to their impossible prepregnancy bodies. We even tell ourselves, in our confusion about what we should expect postpartum, something along the lines of, "if I could just get myself back to what I was before, then everything will be okay." The social pressure to get back to the hot, sexy, non-mom self is enormous. The turbulence caused by the transition into motherhood is real, and yet, we are left totally without any guidance as to how we are to restore ourselves after such a tremendous body and life altering experience.

When you think about what you learned about preparing your body to recover postpartum, what were you told? Is this something your doctor brought up with you? Did your mother, sisters, aunts, or girlfriends share their stories with you in a helpful and positive way that showed you what your game plan should look like? Did anyone help give you perspective on what you should expect for the period of time immediately following the birth around your body, your hormones, your sex life, and your relationship? If any discussion was there, it likely mirrored the conversation around your first period: expect and accept an unavoidable and unchangeable negative physical experience.

So much of the time we use during pregnancy is dedicated to preparing the nursery, planning the baby shower, trying to find clothes that fit your changing body, and dealing with all of the unexpected things that can happen with our bodies, health, and moods during pregnancy, all while making sure you are doing your very best to eat and take care of yourself for the benefit of your baby. It is presented to us as a finite adventure (filled with shopping), which after the birth is then complete. We're encouraged to put so much careful thought and planning into the shower, the nursery, the birth plan. We don't get any guidance on the planning we should be doing to care for the body of the mother who just completed the herculean task of 3-D printing a tiny human for nine months!

We go through the intense, physical experience of delivering that tiny human out into the world safely. We then continue to nourish from our own bodies and nurture that new person with so much intensity and focus. All of this is incredibly depleting of micronutrient stores, and has real impact on the organs, tissues, and fascia of the abdomen, back, and urogenital system. And yet we are left surprised and vulnerable when our health and bodies start to suffer.

This missing conversation not only downplays the largesse of this experience as women, but also undermines our chances of proper recovery. Motherhood is a process of becoming, transforming, and responding, which develops over time and begins in pregnancy. The birth moment is one part of the transformation, but it continues in the fourth trimester and beyond. Yet the support, access to information, and expectations around what is actually needed postpartum leaves much to be desired. What if you were told instead that your pregnancy time is already preparing you emotionally, spiritually, and physically for your transformation into motherhood, and that specific care in the days immediately following the birth are required for your hormonal recovery, your emotional and physical wellbeing both short and long term, and for your ability to be fully present and enjoy the gift of motherhood?

As a functional nutritionist and hormone expert, I've spent the past seventeen years helping women balance their hormones with food, recover from frustrating and debilitating menstrual disturbances like PCOS, fibroids, endometriosis, PMS, and improve their fertility to become the mothers they want to be. Every woman I've ever spoken with, who has long suffered with symptoms and the conventional failed approaches of medication, surgeries, and synthetic hormone replacement, wishes she had been taught how her body worked and how to deal with her inevitable hormonal fluctuations naturally. As someone who has suffered personally with a hormonal imbalance, I know how reclaiming hormonal health totally transforms every aspect of one's life. That is why I wrote *WomanCode*. I wanted there to be a guide for women to navigate the inevitable hormonal turbulence that comes with puberty, periods, pregnancy, postpartum, and peri-menopause, so women everywhere could know what I discovered in my research, that foods, not pharmaceuticals, are the way to restore balance and reclaim your vitality, and that an ongoing relationship with your body and organizing your self-care around the innate cyclical patterns of your biochemistry is the only way for women to live their healthiest, happiest lives.

Kimberly Johnson leveraged the protocol in *WomanCode* to help regain her hormonal balance during her own postpartum healing process. In her book, she is now sharing all of her vast knowledge as a doula and pelvic floor expert to help women understand how to use this postpartum period as a time to partner deeply with our bodies to reclaim our health and set ourselves up for lifelong wellness as mothers. She will encourage you to listen to your intuition that you do in fact need more support and your own body deserves attention after baby because a healthy mother is best for baby.

When I was preparing to go through my own pregnancy and postpartum, because of my professional training, I knew I needed to assemble a team of support, stock my freezer and pantry, create space in my career for rest, and monitor myself and symptoms closely. I spent the majority of the third trimester putting this together and preparing myself emotionally and physically for the epic journey ahead. This is not a standard way to think of the process, simply because from the earliest moments we are handed a set of beliefs about our bodies; rather, we believe that we are victims to them, that nothing can be done when things go wrong, that suffering is part of our destiny as women. These beliefs stifle our natural instinct to take action and keep us in a passive relationship with our bodies where we feel like victims and not like the leaders we are meant to be.

The Fourth Trimester is an important book and contribution to the women's health collective library. It is a critical read for every woman planning to become a mother. We don't have adequate terminology to describe the things that happen to us. Even in writing this, the auto-correct doesn't recognize the phrase "postpartum"—everywhere I've typed it, it has the red squiggly line under it! Kimberly makes official this conversation about the existence of the term *fourth trimester*, one that has remained somewhat on the fringes of alternative medicine. It's almost incredulous that it isn't part of our normal lexicon. Think of this book as "What to Expect, after You've Finished Expecting." It will help you deal with the real physical impact that birth can cause, as well as provide you with resources to guide recovery. It's now much more common to hear women expressing desire to have more natural birthing experiences, and it's only logical that we would want to bring that same self-awareness and wellness-based approach to the period right after the birth. This book will help you do that.

Kimberly knows first-hand what happens when we don't have access to this conversation, this perspective, and this practical game plan. Kimberly, after the birth of her own daughter, struggled in many aspects of her health and life, and she suffered alone and found it difficult to find resources to support her. Her arduous journey of physical recovery, however, opened her eyes to the struggle we all have as women to make sense of confusing symptoms from our bodies, to navigate through specialists to find the right care, to even know in the first place to seek care out, and of course to actually recover. Kimberly bravely tells her story of how the fourth trimester opened her eyes to all of this, remade her totally not only as a woman, wife, and mother, but also as patient, student, and guide for other women—she is a midwife for the emergent mother during the fourth trimester.

In very practical and approachable ways, you will be guided on all the things to consider after birth, with the express design of reducing any and all sense of overwhelm and stress. There are charts, lists, and exercises to help you organize everything from food and chores, to your desires and ideas on what you want your experience to be at home, with your partner, and as a mother. Kimberly will guide you expertly to make your optimal post-birth plan. She brings real talk around what to expect in healing physically from pregnancy and birth, and this candor extends to preparing for the impact of the birth on your emotions, sex life, and relationship, as well as giving guidance on how to navigate those waters successfully. The more you read this book, the more you will feel encouraged that you are capable of leading yourself and your family through this transition. This is truly what motherhood requires of you: to emerge as a leader.

Kimberly is committed to your well-being as a woman and as a mother. This book is the result of that devotion and love. It emerged from her own commitment to loving herself enough to take care of herself properly and daring to want more for her own health and life. She has laid the trail clear for you, lit the torches, and left you snacks along the way to help you continue the journey, not back to your old self, but out beyond who you've ever known yourself to be before, into the field of motherhood, centered in your own body and with a new and increased confidence in yourself and your strength as a woman.

We all take for granted now that every woman should prepare a birth plan. I believe you should also prepare your post-birth plan for the precious and foundational early days of motherhood. With this book, Kimberly has created a guide that will help you restore your body and expand yourself into the role of a lifetime.

—ALISA VITTI, HHC, author of *WomanCode*, founder
The FLO LivingHormone Center, creator of The MyFLO App

the *fourth* trimester

introduction

.... ✻ ....

Most women expect birth to be a reckoning.

So we prepare for it. We interview doulas, attend childbirth-education classes, choose our care providers carefully, stop eating sushi, and take better care of ourselves than ever before. There are so many books out there, and an endless stream of commentary, on how to best birth a baby; and though it can be overwhelming to sift through all the information, expertise, and personal anecdotes that everyone, from doctors to well-meaning neighbors and perfect strangers, has to offer, we do it enthusiastically—or if not enthusiastically at least diligently.

Then the baby is born. And when we get home from the hospital or our midwives leave the house, a *new phase of life* has begun.

And typically, no one has told us that the postpartum period is its own reckoning, and so we haven't prepared for it. Our birth books may have had a cursory chapter at the end on the postpartum period, but typically, our libraries and preparation have shifted from what to expect during childbirth to how to raise a baby, with no orientation or guide to this pivotal time in our lives as women.

At this point, our bodies are still changing and, more importantly, healing. We're bonding with our new babies and realizing that our nutrition is just as important but in yet another new way. For some reason, there is a silence about birth injuries and how to truly care for ourselves during this time. Most women know to keep an eye out for symptoms of postpartum depression, but beyond that, we may not know much else.

This book aims to fill that gap.

WHAT IS THE FOURTH TRIMESTER?

The *fourth trimester* is a term that describes the three months after your baby is born. Everyone knows that during each trimester of pregnancy, a woman's body changes in rapid and significant ways, and there is a symbiotic relationship between mother and baby. What many women don't know is that the three months after your baby is born are just as important as the earlier three trimesters. You need at least as much if not more attention and care as you did when your baby was in the womb. And when we respect our real and unique needs during the fourth trimester, we set ourselves up for a return to radiant health. Unfortunately, the opposite is also true. When we don't have adequate information and support, we set ourselves up for a long road of dis-ease and recovery.

I, too, lacked this important information during my motherhood journey: I had prepared for my ideal birth but did zero preparation for the time after. It simply did not occur to me that I would need anything other than my breasts and a few onesies. But I emerged from childbirth with a significant birth injury, and despite being armed with knowledge from my experience as a bodyworker and a yoga teacher, as well as being part of a thriving international holistic community, I was shocked. I struggled to find the resources to understand what was happening to me. Google searches—never a good idea for health concerns—yielded tens of thousands of entries on postpartum depression, but nothing on what to do to prevent it or what might be contributing to it. And truthfully, I felt depressed but knew that it was an outcome of being in so much pain and having so little support, rather than a mental health problem. When told I needed a full surgical pelvic-floor reconstruction, I made a promise not only to heal myself completely without surgery but also to help other women after I did.

I kept thinking, if it was that hard for me to put the puzzle pieces of my own healing process together, how could women with much less of an idea of where to look find the information they needed?

And that question and my journey to answering it is why I trained as a birth doula and now use Structural Integration, Sexological Bodywork, and Somatic Experiencing—the modalities that were instrumental in my own healing—in my women's health-care practice. I specialize in helping women prepare for and recover from birth, and have worked with hundreds of women and birth professionals worldwide to help them heal themselves and put the pieces of their multifaceted postpartum healing together.

Care in the Fourth Trimester: A Revolution

Just as childbirth education has become a standard for most women and couples as a part of pregnancy, postpartum care (which includes self-care and community care) needs to become praxis. Other cultures understand the importance of the fourth trimester. In countries all over the world, from India to Korea, from Turkey to Brazil, rituals and practices are in place to support women and, therefore, relationships and community during this time. Even just one hundred years ago here in the United States, there was a practice of "lying-in," which simply meant supporting women as they rested in the months following birth.

The knowledge of the special requirements for postpartum healing is not new knowledge—but it has been largely forgotten. We currently think that what is a necessity is a luxury, and it's time that we reclaim this knowledge for ourselves and for each other, so that rather than feeling depleted, frazzled, and fragile, women can emerge from the transition to motherhood stronger, happier, and more whole.

We live in exciting times. We are in the midst of an awakening to the importance of supporting women and couples in the transition to motherhood and family life. The 2016 presidential election was the first where maternity and paternity leave were mentioned as important campaign issues. Influential companies like Facebook and Microsoft have adopted parental-leave policies of up to four months, replacing the standard six-week maternity leave for women and acknowledging the importance of partner leave. Ten years ago, no one had heard of a doula; now many women wouldn't think of giving birth without one.

I look forward to a time, hopefully not too far away, when women and the mother-baby unit are cared for and revered as a matter of course. Until then, it's important for each woman to fully engage in the process of eliciting her authority: there is no one right way to be pregnant, to give birth, to be a mother. There are as many ways to walk this path as there are women in this world. But when we are surrounded by a web of support and information, we are free to explore what works for ourselves, our babies, and our families.

That is why I have decided to write this book—to give more women the knowledge, tools, and even the permission to find the right postpartum path for themselves. We don't need to wait for company policies and governmental mandates to change. Pregnant women can plan for the postpartum experience that they need and deserve. New moms can find a context to understand why they are feeling what they are feeling, and they can learn sound guiding principles to optimize their experience; and women who care for other women in this phase of life will find in this book a multidimensional tool to supplement their expertise.

HOW TO USE THIS BOOK

This book is designed so you can pick it up and quickly flip to a five- or ten-minute practice, read another woman's story, or browse to find the answer to a lingering question.

Don't worry—you don't have to have any prior experience with yoga, meditation, or bodywork to engage in the exercises. If you do have yoga experience, don't skip over the "simpler" movements. Even if you are familiar with them or they seem too easy, you will experience a faster and more lasting recovery if you are willing to move slowly, step by step, in these first months after birth.

Each chapter concludes with a summary that captures the main ideas; you can return to these again and again. Each chapter also offers reflections, questions, and practices so you can engage with the material and it can become as useful and relevant to your life as possible. This book is a guide, so knowing the information without using it will only go so far. Small, daily investments of time will be a boon toward your postpartum healing and the integration of motherhood into your identity.

Part 1: Preparing for the Fourth Trimester

If you are pregnant, begin with the first section of this book, "Preparing for the Fourth Trimester," which begins with chapter 1, "The Postpartum Revolution." In the first section, I share ways that you can prepare yourself, your household, and your relationship so your postpartum period is as tranquil, even as blissful, as possible. You will craft a postpartum sanctuary plan that helps you anticipate your physical, emotional, and relationship needs after giving birth, and you will assemble your support team, so you know who and how to ask for help when you need it.

You will also find movement exercises in this section that will carry you through birth, guiding you to sensations and reference points you can refer to after you give birth. You will train your nervous system to be resilient and manage stress. Invest just five or ten minutes a day into preparing, and you will reap huge benefits.

In addition to sharing other women's stories and exercises in every chapter, there is also a sample grocery list and a note for your door in the appendices, and resources in the bibliography.

Part 2: Savoring the Fourth Trimester

If you recently had a baby, you can jump right into this section if you like. It begins by reviewing the foundations of health in the postpartum period, which were covered more in depth in chapter 2. (If you want the full exploration or a refresher on the need for postpartum care, feel free to flip back to chapter 1.)

"Savoring the Fourth Trimester" offers a guide to gracefully traversing this important transition and critical period in a new mother's life. Many cultures protect the mother-baby unit during this time, which, in Ayurveda, India's traditional healing modality, is called the *sacred window*. It is an opportunity to strengthen the immune system of both mother and baby, and set the tone of your health and healing to come. This part offers ways to relish the sacred window and elicit support so you can heal now instead of doing repair work later.

I share a week-by-week movement schedule that can be practiced daily until your six-week post-birth visit with your doctor or midwife, outline the hormones that are at play after you give birth, and discuss how to support yourself when surfing the inevitable waves of emotion and change. I take a primarily holistic perspective and offer wisdom from traditional Chinese medicine and Ayurveda, but also include insights from research-based physical therapy and Western medicine's allopathic methods. If you have had birth or recovery complications, this section also addresses many medical realities and how you can work with them to support your short- and long-term health, offering practical ways to explore your birth story, to stay connected to your partner, and to pave the way toward deeper intimacy. Again, other women's stories and exercises, as well as informative sidebars, are sprinkled throughout.

If you feel like you are in the weeds and don't have the support you need, you may want to backtrack to chapter 3, "Creating Your Postpartum Sanctuary Plan." Yes, even if you're already postpartum, building that plan and putting parts of it into action will be integral to restoring your health and vitality.

Part 3: Beyond the Fourth Trimester

The fourth trimester passes, but the process of becoming a mother continues. Part 3 guides you in navigating your evolving new normal. We can never go back to who we were, but we can identify and honor our deeply held values. This is where we discover the mother we are, distinct from how we were mothered. It is also where we confront our ideals, acknowledge realities, and learn what it means to be a "good enough" mother. With so many bodily changes and new identities, this section also guides women through the mysterious process of finding new doorways into their desires and their sexuality.

To bring this process full circle, women are led through how to create their own postpartum ritual, gather community, and share the richness of the journey; they are also encouraged to write their own child a letter, offering the wisdom they have gleaned thus far and claiming this liminal time as worthy of documentation.

OUR JOURNEY INTO MOTHERHOOD

This book is my offering to every woman becoming a mother. It's the book that I desperately wish I'd had. My hope is that it provides the tools, information, encouragement, and comfort you need to make this precious transition smoother. If you are feeling confused, depressed, rearranged, or in pain, may this book serve as an oasis in the desert. I have been where you are, and my sincere hope is that you can find something here that makes sense to you. May you find solace and hope in the stories of other women here, may you find the strength to take one small step out of the darkness, and may your journey be full and rich. Even though you may struggle, even though you may be exhausted, may you also discover inner gems that you didn't even know existed through the power of the love that has been awakened in you.

My Own Birth and
Postpartum Experience

I don't know how much time has passed. It's getting dark again and I am alone. The contractions are getting stronger, and I can't believe there is no one here with me as I am giving birth. I am naked and without my glasses. I pace my apartment, making sure that every corner of the place is safe. Like an animal stalking prey, I want to know where everyone and everything is. I am hyperaware of every smell and every sound that enters this space, but no one is here.

The midwife left around lunchtime, and now the sun is setting. At last, she is back, four hours later, apologizing for abandoning me. But I am already in a hazy other world, a distant land of pacts between my baby and me. We are doing this thing by ourselves, I've decided. We are a team—the two of us against the world. We can do this.

After four more hours of pushing, I birthed my baby girl with raw determination. I did not relax so she could slide out. Pregnant for a long forty-two weeks and five days, and in labor long enough to see the sun rise, set, and then nearly rise again, I had run out of patience. I experienced no birth orgasm, no fetal ejection reflex. I was in my ideal birth setting, and yet the experience was not ideal. Instead, I pushed my daughter out with sheer force, tearing severely, although I didn't feel it at the time.

My first inkling that all was not right was when I realized that the midwives were still between my legs after I had birthed the placenta. Soon I felt the sting of local anesthesia and the tugging of stitches as they repaired the floor of my pelvis. Dread overcame me: I was well aware of the physical, structural, and energetic functions of the pelvic floor, and to have mine severely damaged would predispose me to all kinds of instability and weakness, as well as dysfunction that could take a lifetime to heal. I could be irreparably misshapen and damaged.

What I didn't know was that this was the beginning of one of the biggest and most important healing journeys of my life.

THE ASCENT BEFORE BIRTH

The year before giving birth, I had landed a dream job teaching yoga at a detox spa on an island in Brazil. Living on this island had been like living in a giant womb of pulsing life-force energy and salt water. When I arrived on Ilha Grande, the Big Island, seventy miles south of Rio de Janeiro, I did not have a strong idea of what the feminine was, but the island began to wake her up in me. I hiked barefoot and sometimes naked. I swam in the ocean every day. I lived with hair wet from waterfalls or the sweat of deep yoga practice and passionate lovemaking—the island found a way to seep inside me. The wild one in me had awakened.

Naturally, I fell madly in love with a gorgeous Brazilian man who lived there. I prayed to the Goddess of the sea, Iemanja, to show me what my path was with this man and with Brazil. Within two months, I was pregnant and thrilled.

Without a doubt I was living in a whirlwind of radical changes, but I have always been a cliff diver, and I prepared and planned for the birth exhaustively. I respected birth like I respect the ocean—I knew it was bigger and more powerful than I could fathom. I also arrived at the altar of birth without believing any of the well-meaning friends and students (notably not mothers) who chorused, "Birth will be easy for you because you are so in touch with your body. You're a yogi! You know how to breathe." I taught yoga, including prenatal yoga, but I intuitively knew that the words *birth* and *easy* didn't have any business being in the same sentence.

Yet as humbled and reverent as I was at the altar of birth, like many women, I was naive about what would happen afterward. I was absolutely unaware of what the fourth trimester would require from me or how deeply I would be transformed by it.

It was true that as a longtime yoga practitioner, teacher trainer, and Structural Integration bodyworker, I was already an expert on the pelvic floor, both my own and others'. I was deeply connected to my body, so I couldn't imagine why it would fail me now. After years of voraciously exploring the body-mind connection through dance, yoga, Rolfing, Feldenkrais, and many other forms of therapy, I was absolutely confident in my body's innate wisdom and resiliency.

I had worked through body dysmorphia issues as a young dancer, so I did not expect to feel any kind of estrangement toward my body's changing shape and functions during something as natural as becoming a mother. I had always spent a lot of time around babies and children, so I was confident that I could care for a newborn. I was not concerned that my husband worked nights and slept during the days. I was not worried at all that the only help I would have after the baby came was one week with my mom and one week with my mother-in-law. Like so many new mothers, I was completely unprepared, blind to the other birth that was happening: the birth of myself as a mother.

My fall—from the heights of this ecstatic island love affair to a lonely city apartment where I eventually gave birth—was long. I never imagined that after fulfilling so much of my heart's desire I would end up with a birth that needed healing. It was hard to wrap my mind around the idea that childbirth, which happens nearly 400,000 times per day worldwide, would take such an enormous toll on my body, mind, and spirit.

THE FALL

After giving birth, my reality shifted dramatically. The simple act of walking was so painful that for months I couldn't make it to the grocery store. I would just not eat until someone went to the store for me. For two months, I wasn't able to sit. It took more than two years for the constant lower back pain, hemorrhoids, and searing pain during sex to ease up. This was all a far cry from the invincible mothers I saw bouncing right back—the woman at the pool with her five-day-old, the CEOs returning to work days after giving birth, the fellow yoga teachers back in the yoga studio a month after giving birth, not to mention my own self-image as a hotshot, young yoga teacher and bodyworker.

I also had no idea that being away from my roots, the women in my family—sister, mother, grandmother, and dear, familiar friends—would have such an impact on my ability to heal after the birth. Nor did I imagine how going nearly three weeks past my due date, pushing for such a long time during labor, and sustaining a significant tear would affect my ability to recover. Individually these elements would have required significant healing, but together they more than tripled my healing time.

As disheartening as my symptoms were, I was even more perplexed by the lack of resources available to assist my healing. My midwives were either too busy, at a loss for how to help, or in denial about the severity of my situation to assist me in any real way.

On the Internet, I found thousands of entries on how to identify postpartum depression. But my situation seemed much more complex than a simple label could explain. It was not surprising that I was depressed after ten months of ongoing physical, emotional, and spiritual issues, not to mention the practical and cultural challenges I faced every day. I was limited by my language skills and by cultural misunderstandings, unsure if postpartum resources simply didn't exist in Brazil, or if I just didn't know where to look. It felt like my body was falling apart, and I had no resources to help myself, plus I had spent my life savings to hire a midwife I trusted and to have the birth I wanted. I had no childcare options, so I couldn't work. My partner was well meaning but as unprepared as I was, and often absent.

THE SEARCH

My trusted healers, acupuncturists, osteopaths, and pelvic-floor physical therapists were all in the United States. I was conflicted about leaving Brazil without my husband, who would need to go through a Byzantine system of paperwork to be allowed to enter the country, but I was running out of options.

So, leaving my husband behind in Rio, I flew with my daughter to Boulder, Colorado, where many of my contacts were. My first stop was an obstetrician for a checkup on my pelvic floor. Although I tend to approach allopathic medical protocols cautiously, I wanted a straight-up evaluation from someone who would not sugarcoat it. I was still finding feces in my underpants without even having had the urge to go, experiencing unbearable pain during sex, and enduring constant sacral and lower back dysfunction that made me grab my back every time I stood up and sat down.

Upon hearing my long list of symptoms—but not examining me—the obstetrician recommended full pelvic floor reconstructive surgery. Knowing that the pelvic floor was the root of spinal health, organ health, and energetic connection to the earth, the last thing I wanted was to be cut open and then knitted back together with materials my body would not recognize. I knew only too well that surgery didn't always solve things, and, in fact, sometimes complicated them. This was not just a pelvic floor—this was a sacred opening and passageway. My response was: no way.

As I walked out of the office, I was even more determined to understand what I was going through. If I, with all my bodywork and yoga experience, could not find the resources I needed to fully recover from birth without surgery, how could the average woman get the help she needed? What I sought was a multifaceted approach to healing that would take into account these layers of experience in my very real and complex transition to motherhood.

So began my transition from free spirit to feet-on-the-ground seeker. I was determined. I made an appointment with my holistic pelvic-floor health specialist, Michele Kreisberg, and as our visit approached, I anxiously anticipated hearing more bad news. Happily, Michele told me that there was a lot of healing available before resorting to surgery. And just knowing that I wasn't a hopeless case gave me the energy to continue pursuing natural healing.

After living in Boulder for several months, I needed the support of my family. I returned to San Diego to live with my parents so I could continue to care for my daughter full-time. I hoped that my husband would soon join us. I sought out my longtime yoga teachers and colleagues, but every time I practiced—even at basic levels—my back pain and the incontinence and hemorrhoids worsened. I continued with the remedial physical therapy exercises and experimented with physical exercises I could do that strengthened rather than weakened me.

Six months later, a little more healed thanks to the consistent, gentle practices, and finally able to teach, I received a job offer to colead a yoga teacher training in Thailand. I was eager to investigate age-old Asian traditions of protecting and caring for women in the early months after birth. I also knew that in Thailand I would be able to afford full-time childcare and dedicate my extra time to my own healing process. Up until that point, like many new mothers, I had tended to sacrifice my own basic needs to attend to my daughter's.

After living in the United States without my husband for a year, my now almost-two-year-old daughter and I set off for Asia.

LESSONS IN HEALING

At the teacher training, the universe sent me an angel in the form of Ellen Heed, a sexological bodyworker who taught the anatomy portion of the program. Sexological Bodywork is a progressive, holistic field that includes the treatment of sexual and reproductive anatomy in its scope of practice. When I got up the courage to tell her about my symptoms, she invited me to participate in a groundbreaking study she was conducting with postpartum moms and scar-tissue remediation. Through my sessions with her, my incontinence, hemorrhoids, and a diastasis (a separation in my abdominal wall)—the conditions the doctor in Boulder had been certain would require comprehensive surgery—healed. It seemed like a miracle.

Now that I was turning my attention to my own healing, I carved out time to reflect on everything that had happened in the last two years. I made it a project to face the disappointment and grief over the loss of my yoga practice as I knew it, my sovereignty over my body, and my dream of a traditional family. My marriage, I finally admitted to myself, was coming apart.

I now saw that I had married a man who I'd always known was an unlikely match for me. We had nothing in common—neither language nor socioeconomic background nor life trajectory. What we had was a pure and innocent bond that I had hoped would be enough to support a life together in sync with the rhythms of the rainforest. After a year of waiting, I had to nod to the intuition I had felt from the first time I met him that he was an island boy at heart, who would never leave Brazil.

When the monthlong teacher training was complete, I decided to stay in Thailand to enjoy the lower cost of living and slower pace of life. Each day, after I'd dropped my daughter off at preschool, I would lie down on the cold tile in our small guesthouse to let my emotions come, washing over me and sinking in. Then I'd do a short yin yoga practice and pray. Late nights, I turned my full attention to building a website and a viable business, and to envisioning a future for me and my daughter.

Giving birth and becoming a mother had reshaped me. I did not want other women to suffer from the same lack of resources and wisdom that I had grappled with after I gave birth. My deepest wounds have always become my greatest teachers, and this was no exception. I began to hear the call to serve new mothers and try to fill what felt like a black hole in women's health—the postpartum period.

Determined to broaden my vision of women's health and fill in the gaps in my understanding of holistic postpartum healing while in Asia, I sought out perspectives from as many modalities and cultures as I could.

Thailand is strongly influenced by Chinese culture and medicine, so I decided to start my research exactly where I was. I interviewed women and healers about how women were cared for during the postpartum period. I even found a center that hired out massage therapists and herbalists to new mothers. The healers went to women's houses every day for forty days with special recipes, herbs, and wraps to help assist them through the transition to motherhood. Friends from Korea and Hong Kong spoke of a "confinement period" during which new mothers were cared for and served special soups to aid them in healthy recovery.

I recalled India, where new mothers return to their own mothers' home after giving birth to be fed, sponge bathed, and kept calm as she got to know her baby. I felt the importance of the matrilineal wisdom traditions—generations of women helping out—and extended family, and for the first time understood the impact of my choice to give birth outside of my motherland, away from my own lineage. I had been unprotected at a time when I was meant to be sheltered and surrounded. I had had no comfort food, no familiar smells, and no comforting sights or companions. I had been fending for myself when I should have been leaning on the support of my friends and family.

A CALL TO HELP OTHERS HEAL

When my daughter and I finally returned to California, I decided to train as a birth doula so I could support other women in their passage from conception through childbirth to motherhood. As I began to integrate what I had learned about pelvic health and scar tissue into my bodywork practice, women sought me out to address specific birth-related health problems. In some cases, these issues had begun for them during childbirth and had gone unresolved for up to twenty years. Some of these problems we were able to resolve in just one session.

At this point, I had been away from Brazil for a year and a half. My daughter was no longer speaking Portuguese. Her father spoke no English. If she was going to have a relationship with her father and to her roots, I needed to take her back to Brazil. I owed it to my daughter to honor her roots and give her a chance to connect to her birthplace and her father.

So, my daughter and I returned to Brazil in November 2009. I was determined to focus my work on helping expat women navigate their birth experiences in Brazil and to making a difference in the community of advocates for safe, healthy, and woman-centered births, called "humanized birth." Brazil has an 80 percent cesarean rate, one of the highest cesarean section rates in the world, so I knew there was a lot of work to do.

In my subsequent years in Rio, I accompanied dozens of women from countries as far away as Cape Verde and Australia as they went through conceptions, miscarriages, pregnancies, births, and postpartum experiences of all kinds. The roles I played were diverse too: from yoga teacher to medical translator, to childbirth educator, birth doula, and, eventually, practitioner of Somatic Experiencing, a form of therapy that addresses the impact of trauma on the nervous system and is a perfect complement to hands-on healing.

MAGAMAMA

From all my training, advocacy, and hands-on work, I became known affectionately in my bohemian Rio neighborhood of Santa Teresa as the *maga*, which means "sorceress" in Portuguese. But it was really my work with these inspiring women that showed me all women are magas, and to become a mother is to become an alchemist, balancing multiple roles and identities, often journeying to the underworld and back. The stories I heard and lived revealed women's hidden strength, power, and magic, awakened through the transformative power of birth.

Today, women from all over the world—from Sweden to Spain to Korea—contact me for online consultations and in-person healing sessions regarding their birth stories, birth injuries, trauma, and healing. Women's stories reinforce that it was not just my particular experience as an American living abroad in an unconventional relationship that made my postpartum period difficult. Women everywhere are experiencing difficulty adapting to motherhood. According to the New York State Department of Health, as many as 80 percent of women say that they experience "baby blues" after giving birth. And as I knew all too well, in some cases, postpartum depression is a result of the convergence of a complex set of personal and cultural circumstances, rather than strictly a women's mental health problem.

In 2014, my daughter and I moved back to my hometown, San Diego, where I set up a private practice. It had taken nearly seven years, but I once again had access to my full life force and was able to use my body without fear of injury. I returned to a deep network of support that included my parents and my sister and that I could lean into. I completed training in Sexological Bodywork, and in my clinic, I combine hands-on, hands-in work, with Birth Story Medicine and body-centered therapy to help women feel whole again after childbirth. I bridge the worlds of birth, sex, and trauma. Each day I assure women that what they are feeling is normal, that they are not "behind" in their healing process, and that they are not alone.

After years of working on this book project, I finally had the depth of support that I needed to birth it and to grow it! This book is my offering to you—the book I wish I had when I was becoming a mother. Motherhood, like no other life experience, has shown me clearly and profoundly how interconnected our physical, mental, emotional, and spiritual health is.

This was my heroine's journey. It was long and arduous—longer and more arduous than most. I am not who I was. I am someone new. While the circumstances of your life may be less extreme than mine were (and I truly hope that they are!), I hope that my story will serve as a torch for your own journey. When you give birth, it is not just your baby that is born; in a way, you are born. This is a profound and glorious birth itself—your birth as a mother. All births require celebration, treasuring, and deep care. The liminal space between stages of life is delicate. While there are normal difficulties and challenges that every new mother faces, when the path is lit by those who have gone before us, there is the possibility of making the transition with grace and ease.

May your motherhood journey be filled with richness, depth, and insight!

Part One

PREPARING FOR THE
FOURTH TRIMESTER

.... ❧ ....

Don't forget love; it will bring all the madness
you need to unfurl yourself across the universe.
—MIRABAI

While there's a good chance you've been preparing for your baby's birth by reading books, taking birthing classes, and preparing your home, you may not be preparing yourself for the changes that *you* will be experiencing. You have probably carefully chosen who you want at your birth to support you, what you want the birth environment to feel like, and how you will be able to get what you need so you can have the birth you want. But if you are anything like me, you probably haven't thought much about what it will be like when the birth is over.

Sure, you might have considered how you want to care for your baby. Many women have considered what kind of nourishment they want to give their babies (breastfeeding, formula, bottle feeding, and so on), investigated sleep philosophies, or even taken an infant-care class. We make room in our lives for our babies—in our homes, in our daily routines, in regard to our work lives—but somehow we forget just how much and how rapidly our own bodies and identities are going to change.

If you're approaching giving birth, this section will help you prepare, not for the birth itself—I'm sure you have plenty of resources and support for that—but for what will come directly after. This journey is an invitation to discover deeper levels of your inner world—your strengths, your vulnerabilities, your beliefs. Welcome to this sacred journey of motherhood.

··· 1 ···

the postpartum revolution

It is one of the most complex and interesting times in history to be a woman and to be a mother. We are rife with choices, inundated by them. We can craft our own lives. We can be breadwinners while our partners stay home. We can be astronauts; we can be homemakers. We can work from home. We can almost be president. We are not tied to a single location. We can live far away from our families and our work. We can eat pineapple and mangos in winter. We can be anywhere in the world in under two days. We can call people and see their faces through video almost anywhere in the world. Through social media, we have a perception of closeness and connection. In some ways, we have ultimate freedom. In others, we are suffering more than ever.

What is natural has become countercultural. What is necessity is now considered luxury. What is luxury is considered necessity. What is instinctual is foreign. What should be innate has to be relearned.

We've started to believe that technology is more trustworthy and reliable than nature. We have become accustomed to a level of convenience that makes any discomfort seem abnormal. We are being conditioned to field huge amounts of input and stimuli that make the pace of nature seem painfully slow. We are used to having what we want the moment we want it.

The idea of the fourth trimester that includes a period of forty days spent resting, nurturing ourselves, and letting others nurture us, challenges our deeply held cultural tropes of individualism and self-sufficiency, some of our feminist ideals, and our personal expectations that we are unstoppable superwomen. The fourth trimester goes unrecognized as an important part of women's health care.

In all my years of spiritual practice, I never experienced anything that showed me the interconnection of all that makes us human and makes up true radiant wellness like I did during the postpartum process. I had to attend to every level of my self—physical, mental, emotional, sexual, and spiritual—to come back to total health.

Yet, for all of its potential power, this period of time is overlooked. Doctors and midwives provide little information. After methodically preparing for birth, women are left to figure out the monumental transition to becoming a mother on their own. At a time when women need more support than ever, we are left isolated, wondering what happened, who we are, and what we can do about it.

No wonder as many as 15–20 percent of women experience postpartum depression. In the absence of conversation about how we can care for ourselves and be cared for when we become mothers, and in the absence of dialogue about women's health over a lifetime, this issue is often reduced to a women's mental health problem alone.

If you have a baby, you will experience the postpartum period. It is a stage of life—a wonderfully and mystifyingly transformative period in a new mother's life that doesn't have to lead to depression. While the landscape may seem grim, the good news is that cultures all over the world have a roadmap for supporting women through this transition, and it's pretty simple. But let's build this from the ground up. First, what exactly is the fourth trimester?

WHAT EXACTLY IS THE POSTPARTUM PERIOD?

"How long is this going to last?" is the question most frequently asked by women who come to my office. I too had that same question.

Is it nine days? Six weeks? Three months? Nine months? Two years? Forever?

About a year after my daughter was born, still in the throes of my own issues (as mentioned above in my birth and postpartum story), I asked one of my wise mother friends how long "all this" was going to last, meaning feeling physically, emotionally, and spiritually reconfigured. When was I going to feel put back together again? When could I expect to recognize myself?

Her answer was ten years.

At the time, it floored me. Looking back, I think it was one of the most candid, realistic and, eventually, soothing pieces of good sense that I received. How could I expect anything less from such a considerable overhaul that included a life-force transfer, a totally identity shift, and a physical rearrangement?

Ten years was certainly a far cry from what I'd read in magazine features about actresses and high-powered executives returning to work after two weeks. My yoga teacher friends, too, were back in the studio as early as one or two months after giving birth. An acquaintance whom I saw at the pool each day was swimming up until the day she gave birth, and when I saw her five days later in the pool, I did a double take. Where was her baby? How was she already back swimming?

All around us is the message: *Get your body back. Get back into a routine. Get back into your prepregnancy jeans.* And those are just the overt messages, which are so prevalent for new mothers. The underlying message is to get through this period as fast as possible; return to the familiar; return to what you recognize and what you know.

Thinking longer term—*much* longer term—allowed me to take the pressure off. I could stop feeling like there was something wrong with me for not feeling normal sooner. For the hundreds of new mothers I have worked with in my office and taught in workshops, the persistent questions are: Why doesn't anyone talk about this? When will I feel like myself again? When will postpartum be over?

Average Maternity Leave in the United States

The Family and Medical Leave Act (FMLA) states that some businesses (all public agencies, all public and private elementary and secondary schools, and companies with fifty or more employees) must provide eligible employees with up to twelve weeks of unpaid leave each year for the birth and care of a newborn child. But according to the Bureau of Labor and Statistics, only 12 percent of Americans have access to paid parental leave, which means there's a lot of people out there who don't qualify for paid leave. And according to the Center for Economic and Policy Research, two in five women do not qualify, and the Department of Labor found that 64 percent of eligible women and 36 percent of eligible men don't take it.

What does that all mean? First and foremost, it means that most Americans are not able to take off from work after having a baby. About 25 percent of American women go back to work *ten days* after giving birth.

According to figures from the National Center for Health Statistics, about two-thirds of U.S. women are employed during pregnancy, and about 70 percent of them report taking some time off. How much time? Well, the average maternity leave for American women is about ten weeks, while about half of new moms took at least five weeks and about a quarter took nine weeks or more.

Defining *Postpartum*

The meaning of the Latin *postpartum* is literally "bringing forth" or "after birth." The very definition drives home the point that, after having a baby, we women are permanently postpartum. We can never return to who and what we were before giving birth. This broader understanding can help you fully absorb how much time it can take to fully integrate all the changes you go through giving birth and becoming a mother.

Beyond this general definition, the postpartum period can be defined in many ways. Some definitions limit the postpartum period from nine to eleven days, when the uterus returns to its prepregnancy size. Many cultures share the idea of a *golden month*, or confinement period, that is anywhere from twenty to sixty days, and often around forty days.

In India and Japan, a new mother goes back to her own mother's house for six weeks, so she is relieved of all household duties—cooking, cleaning, and caring for her husband. In China, duties are split between mother and mother-in-law; new moms are supported in sitting out the month, so they can regain their physical vitality and strength. One client of mine shared that her El Salvadoran mother-in-law came all the way to California from the East Coast for the birth of both my client's children, insisting that my client honor the first forty days after giving birth.

Some definitions of the *postpartum period* include the completion of the fourth trimester. Others consider the period to be nine months, the age when human babies reach the stage of development that other mammal babies are already at when they are born. In still another definition, two years, the age it is commonly recommended to wean a baby at, is the demarcation of the end of the postpartum phase.

Here in the United States, what marks many women's postpartum experiences is the six-week post-birth doctor visit. The timing mirrors the older wisdom of the immediate postpartum period; however, this visit is usually so short and superficial that women are left thinking, *That's it? A quick exam and I'm free to return to exercise and work. Okay, but HOW? Everything's "normal," but I don't really feel normal.*

There is no clear consensus on exactly how long this period lasts, which makes sense, because the process that each woman goes through after giving birth is unique. The length of the postpartum period is different for every woman, but it is almost universally longer than we want it to be, expect it to be, and think it should be.

When we remember that the postpartum period seems longer than we think it should be, perhaps we can give ourselves a break. We can adjust our expectations, and instead of insisting on our familiar, faster pace, we can soften into a slower rhythm, so we can truly relish what this time has to offer. Rather than minimizing it or trying to get through it as quickly as possible, we can decelerate, be present, and even savor the experience. You may be thinking, *Sure, that sounds amazing, but how?* It starts with the knowledge of the roadmap that is shared across cultures and honors the five universal needs of all postpartum women everywhere.

FIVE UNIVERSAL POSTPARTUM NEEDS

There are remarkable similarities in the ways that women are cared for all around the world after they give birth. While specifics may differ, what is shared across cultures is the attention to creating an environment that respects the five universal postpartum needs. Those needs are:

- an extended rest period;
- nourishing food;
- loving touch;
- the presence of wise women and spiritual companionship; and
- contact with nature.

Extended Rest Period

Around the world, new mothers are expected to rest for the first twenty to sixty days after giving birth. Women are literally sequestered in order to rest. Women are cared for so that they can direct all their care toward their babies. A new mother is supported in resting so as to give her body, mind, and spirit time to harmonize and process everything she has just experienced. Both classical Chinese medicine and Ayurveda—the two modalities that offered me the most healing support—view this time as the most critical in ensuring a woman's long-term health.

The Chinese call this period *zuo yuezi*, which means "sitting out the month," sometimes translated as "confinement." I have also heard it referred to as the golden month. In India, this period is called the sacred window, and women move from their marital house back into their mothers' houses so they have no household responsibilities: they know if a woman is in her own house, she won't resist housekeeping! Vietnamese women respect this time called *nằm ổ*, "lying in a nest," by eating tonics and soups, and sitting over charcoal steam prepared by their aunts and mothers. In Mexico and Guatemala, this forty-day rest period for healing and mother-infant bonding is called *la cuarentena*.

This immediate forty-day window postpartum is considered so potent that a woman can heal lifelong illnesses and restore her health, or she can become vulnerable to diseases that take a lifetime to attend to. As noted just above, our modern six-week postpartum health-care checkup is a nod to this knowledge that the six-week mark is a significant moment in the health of mother and baby. Yet it is not accompanied by the intensive nurturing between the birth and the visit itself.

Nourishing Food

Food is a fundamental human need and makes up the building blocks of our body. More importantly, food is medicine. New mothers need special foods during this time. A new mother should consume certain herbs and foods, so she can complete the cleansing of the uterus, eliminate any old blood still remaining, and rebuild her strength. These foods also help a woman to produce milk with more ease. Since a new mother is vulnerable to cold and wind, she needs foods that are both warm in temperature and that have an internal warming effect due to the spices used.

In Hong Kong, women are fed special soups, first for elimination and ease of digestion, and then to rebuild blood and life force. In Korea, soups are made with many kinds of seaweed, which is full of rich minerals. While there are variations in ingredients and spices from culture to culture, what the postpartum foods have in common across cultures is that they are warming, easy to digest, mineral rich, and collagen dense.

Loving Touch

During the birth and postpartum period, women's bodies are going through tremendous changes. Organs are returning to their optimal positions. The body is returning to a normal blood and fluid volume. Hormones are recalibrating. To assist in all these changes, to flush the lymph and to optimize circulation, bodywork is an integral part of a woman's recovery to vibrant health. Because of this understanding, Asian cultures pamper new mothers. In Korea, a new mother gets a massage every day for forty days to help restore organ position and circulation. In India, women receive *abhyanga*, circulatory massage with herbal-infused oils, from sisters and aunts. In Mexico, women are taken through a "closing of the bones" ceremony that includes massage, herbal steam, cathartic release, and being tightly wrapped. In the Indo-Malay tradition, women's bellies are intricately wrapped, and that practice is now also in Singapore, India, Nepal, Taiwan, and Hong Kong too. It's important to have caring touch during this time period, whichever tradition you decide to incorporate into your healing.

Presence of Wise Women and Spiritual Companionship

In most cultures, birth and new motherhood are still considered the territory of women. Therefore, women are surrounded by and tended to by other women who are in different stages of life and who can offer them soul comfort as well as knowledge from experience as aunts, mothers, and grandmothers. There are the practical considerations, such as how to breastfeed, how to care for any small vaginal tears, and what to eat. Then there is the very real fluctuating emotional state, and having other women who have been where you are and can share their experiences is balm to the sensitive heart and nerves.

In many countries, this post-birth time is respected as a delicate one, physically and spiritually, for mothers and babies. In Hopi and Mayan traditions, unmarried and elder women take care of new mothers, so they are relieved of their normal duties and responsibilities and can simply care for their babies during this time. In Turkey, women are kept in the company of loved ones for forty days. The idea is to distract the evil spirits and to keep people from looking directly into the baby's eyes, possibly stealing a part of their spirit. Women need to know that they are not all alone, that they can relax because there are other women around who can care for the home, care for the baby, and care for the mother in this new, vulnerable state.

Contact with Nature

In our high-tech, fast-paced lives, we often forget about the tremendous teacher and resource we have in the natural world. In nature, a seed sprouts, a flower bud blossoms—each process in its own time. We can't force it to happen faster. We can provide the conditions— the right soil, sunlight, and water—for optimal growth, but we cannot push it to happen any faster than its natural rhythm. This is the same in the fourth trimester; life takes on its own pace, one that is entirely unique in its golden languorous quality. Connection to nature can help you feel the beauty and rightness of the slower pace at this time.

It's not necessary to go hiking or camping to feel the power of nature. You can do simple things. Set up a nursing station near a window with a view. Take a sponge bath in warm herbal infusions, as the women do in Mexico, Guatemala, and Brazil. Relish the multilayered flavors of herbal teas. Imbibe the earthy qualities of herbs in your sitz baths and steams. Trade screen time for sitting outside, bundled up, absorbing the feeling of the elements around you. Allow yourself to breathe fully. Feel the air coming into your body, follow its trail and then consciously exchange it back out into the environment. These are all simple ways to reconnect with the elements of nature, the life force around you.

IN CONCLUSION

In places where the culture is not explicitly designed to honor this time immediately after birth, women have to take measures to create their own sanctuaries of relaxation and restoration. At first, the amount of support we need seems surprising, maybe even excessive, especially given the superwoman ideal currently prevalent in the Western world. Women are supposed to give birth and bounce back without missing a beat. Yet the truth is, a new mother needs to be mothered herself, so she can help and effectively learn how to mother her baby.

The five universal postpartum needs are shared across cultures because they follow our physiological design and needs as women. Our investment in this time is an acknowledgement of the preciousness of life—not just the baby's life, but also the mother's life. The postpartum time needs to be recognized as distinct although less obvious than pregnancy. When we skip over this time and do not attend to these needs, we become vulnerable to illness, often an outcome of isolation and loneliness. When we heed the rhythm of this time, we set ourselves up for a smooth transition characterized by interconnectedness and wholeness, where a woman feels the support, wisdom, and presence of her community. When a woman feels supported, the baby thrives, the relationship thrives, our community thrives, and our planet thrives.

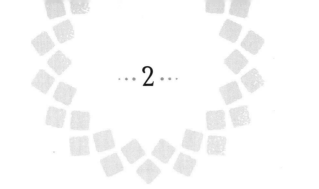

··· 2 ···

setting yourself up
for a smooth transition
to motherhood

While the momentous transition that is giving birth has its unpredictable elements, not the least of which is the uniqueness of the baby that you birth, there are many ways that you can set yourself up to make this transition as smooth as possible, and even thoroughly enjoy it!

It's not always an easy process. After all, having your body, mind, and spirit rearranged is an overhaul that requires the utmost respect and attention. I've been through it, and not just myself, but also with hundreds of women as they navigated conceptions, miscarriages, pregnancies, births, and postpartum experiences of all kinds.

I can attest that preparing the environment you will be recovering in so it nurtures this transition is the first step toward a strong beginning for your family. You will need maturity, foresight, and courage. You'll have to go against what our culture currently says: that a fast recovery will earn you the label of Superwoman. You may be called selfish or spoiled. You may actually feel selfish or spoiled. But it starts here, with honoring the magnitude of what it is to birth a child into the world.

Ideally, this environment is already in place, but because, as a culture, we don't fully recognize how important it is to support women at this time, that may not be true. This isn't to say you don't have a supportive partner, family, friends, and job. You very well may have some or all of those. However, what we're talking about here is different. We're not talking specifically about a loving partner who is excited about the baby and friends who will throw you a shower. We're talking about being sure you and those who already love and support you are prepared for how fully and how long you should rest and be *physically*, as well as emotionally, supported after giving birth.

If you are anything like me, you have done a whole lot of preparation for your baby's birth. Giving birth is a life-altering experience, and it deserves all the care, preparation, planning, and forethought that you have been dedicating to it. But few of us have applied the same questions we asked about childbirth to the postpartum period, such as:

- What support will I need?
- Who do I want to support me and my family during this time?
- What do I want my home to feel like during the immediate postpartum period?
- How will I be able to get my needs met so that, rather than exhausted and depleted, I can emerge stronger and more whole from this transformation?

Make no mistake: any lack of consideration or forethought up to this point is not due to negligence on your part. There is very little, if any, cultural conversation about what the transition to becoming a mother is like for women. When there is conversation, it normally begins after we are already so deep in the postpartum haze that it is hard to see a way back to clarity or to reach out a hand for help.

This chapter seeks to remedy this void and help you anticipate some common after-birth challenges, so you can set yourself up to have an empowering and fulfilling postpartum bonding time with your baby, your partner, and the rest of your family. We'll cover some basic ways to prepare for that period to help you know what to expect and to know what you can do beforehand.

In addition to creating a postpartum sanctuary plan, we will also practice some of the underlying key principles that will allow you to implement and enjoy the plan most effectively. These include learning how to rest, adjusting your expectations, leaning into the feminine, and asking for help.

PREPARING TO REST

My two best friends gave birth a few months before me, each of them going into labor at thirty-six weeks. So at thirty-six weeks, I was thinking that, any day, it could be my turn. I spent my last month of pregnancy going on walks along the beach, eating ice cream—a welcomed mandate from my midwife—loving my partner, and then spending time with my mom, who eagerly showed up on my due date, the forty-week mark. I also slept more than I had ever slept. One night I slept for fourteen hours. (Later, I realized my body was intelligently storing up sleep for birthing and mothering.)

Then came forty-one weeks, then forty-two weeks. I was living in Rio de Janeiro and was already recognized all over town as the pregnant foreigner. I started having dreams about elephant gestation, the longest of all mammals'—elephants carry their young for two years! In my dreams, people were spotting me in different neighborhoods, the redheaded *gringa* who was eternally pregnant. "There she is again, still pregnant, just getting bigger and bigger," they'd say.

In those last weeks of pregnancy, I hauled myself across town on a bus each week to a movement class with pregnant women who shared the same midwife. We all waddled in and did a combination of wrist circles, snakelike belly-dance hip undulations, and woo-

woo visualizations. At the beginning of one of the classes, as we settled in, lying comfortably on the floor, each one of us checked in with a word that represented how we were feeling. Each person chimed in: *alegria*, happiness; *força*, strength; *nervosa*, anxious. Then it was my turn: *preguiçiosa*, lazy. You could hear the group inhale and the *aaaaahhhh*, followed by an enthusiastic, "*Que delicia!*" How delicious!

Huh? I thought. *How delicious?*

Growing up American, I can't think of a single positive connotation with the word *lazy*. Calling someone lazy is the equivalent of calling her or him worthless or a loser in our society. So when the entire room of pregnant mamas and midwives collectively sighed and celebrated my laziness, it gave me pause. Maybe I had something to learn from the idea of laziness being a *good* thing. Maybe I needed to surrender into feeling lazy. Lazy was exactly what a pregnant woman past her due date and living in a tropical climate should be, so why not try to befriend that feeling?

First, we have to be convinced that resting is important. From years of teaching yoga, I have experienced firsthand just how difficult it is for many of us to truly rest and relax. I couldn't tell you how many students have taken my yoga classes and left before the final resting pose, *savasana*. A resting pose seems like a waste of time compared to the active and difficult parts of class, much to the chagrin of this teacher (and most, if not all, of other teachers as well).

Why is it so hard for us to rest? What is going on that it takes so much effort to arrive at a state of non-effort or relaxation? Partially it's a societal problem. We glorify and reward fast-paced, nonstop productivity. Everything from diets to exercise programs promise high-level energy at all times—and we want that. We want to be bulletproof and unstoppable. We want to sleep better, and have better digestion and better birthing experiences, but we don't really want to slow down.

A number of books, articles, and studies in the past decade have touched on this aspect of our lives, coming up with such new terms as *the cult of busyness* and *time poverty*. There are many studies out there that show the effects of stress on our health, but for our purposes here, the biggest issue is that many of us say and think we're busy, but we're not actually as busy as we say we are, at least, according to the U.S. Bureau of Labor Statistics' "American Time Use Survey." And that's a good thing, because it means when we say or think, "There's just not enough time in the day," well, there is. And the fourth trimester is a period in our lives where we should not hesitate to take that time.

But it isn't just an issue with our culture. Sometimes even when we know we want to rest or finally have the time, we can't. We feel anxious or restless, when we are trying to wind down we actually have to learn how to rest. This is because of our bodies' chemistries and rhythms. Without interference, our bodies go through natural cycles of activity and rest, expansion and contraction every day.

These cycles are called *ultradian rhythms*, and they happen about every ninety to one hundred and twenty minutes. We can be active and focused for about ninety minutes. Then we need a five to ten minute period of rest in order to return to optimal brain function for the next cycle.

When we follow this biological rhythm and take a break, we begin the next cycle of activity with brightness and vigor. When we ignore the need to slow down, we often lean on an external source of energy, like caffeine, or we borrow from our own internal reserves of stress hormones, such as adrenaline and cortisol, to push us forward. In doing so, we are overriding our bodies' natural ability to self-regulate, and we are unlearning how to rest.

You can start forming a habit of surfing your ultradian waves of activity and rest right now. The next time it's midmorning or midafternoon and you are feeling a slump in your energy and are about to have a tea or coffee, either do something that will allow your mind to wander or engage your body instead. Instead of ramping yourself up with caffeine, do one of the following:

- go for a five to ten minute, brisk walk;
- lie down on the floor and put your legs up against the wall;
- do some gentle stretching;
- let your eyes wander and daydream; or
- curl up on your side in the fetal position.

Honoring these cycles of activity and rest is a secret not only to having a more productive day, but also to having a more fulfilling birth experience. The idea is to surrender to whatever phase you are in—activity or rest—and simply be in it, not anticipating the next phase. For example, if you are feeling spaced out, unable to focus, or overwhelmed, even if it is not within one of the specific ultradian rhythm cycles—and that happens; we are not robots!—take a few minutes and let your brain recharge. Don't force yourself to push through it. Take a walk. Do a few stretches. Whatever low-energy activity you decide to engage in, stay in it and try to just enjoy it.

This same state of mind goes for later in pregnancy and while you give birth. If you are having a contraction, fully focus and ride that wave. Then, as the surge subsides, notice the tide flow back out during the space between contractions, giving your body the gift of total relaxation. Then there is energy available for the next surge. When you have practiced resting, you can find the space between contractions. Your body will recognize the rest, however brief. Learning to ride waves, rather than plow through them, will serve you in life as well as in the birth and postpartum process.

The Time Directly Before Birth

Even though we may have a desire to go slower, the way most women enter their postpartum period these days is a bit like they are flying down the freeway at high speed—but then they have to hit the brakes and come to a screeching halt. Many of the women I work with, from public defenders to professors to personal trainers, have so little maternity leave that they are forced to choose between time off before birth or after it. Understandably, many women work as close to their due date as possible, so they can use the time to spend it with their babies afterward.

Ideally, all women would have a few weeks before giving birth to shift gears, to downshift and transition smoothly. Not everyone has the lifestyle that I was living, leisurely experiencing the weeks leading up to giving birth. While I do recommend that women give themselves some space to transition from work mind to birthing mind, I realize it is not a viable reality for many women.

If that is the case, that your circumstances mean you have to work down to the wire, it's even more important that you turn your attention to your ultradian rhythms, allowing for small moments of rest during your day, even if you have to go to your car, into the bathroom, or put on noise-canceling headphones with relaxing music. Try the following exercise.

LEARNING TO REST

1. For those of you who already have kids, live with partners, family, or roommates, and all of us who have fast-paced lives: Don't worry. This is only going to be for five minutes. Get up just five minutes earlier, or ask someone at home to time you and help you by doing your duties (loading the dishwasher, watching the kids, etc.) for just five minutes. Tell them they can even time it and you'd actually like them to stop you at the five-minute mark, as this is an exercise.
2. Start by turning off your phone, putting away your laptop, and shutting off the TV or any other electronics.
3. Now go to a quiet room or, if possible, outside.
4. Sit down.
5. Close your eyes if you are not in public and are somewhere you feel safe to do so.
6. Now just sit.

7. This isn't meditating. You don't have to let your thoughts go by and not engage. Engage if you want to, but just sit. Get used to what it feels like *not* to have someone demanding something from you, or some electronic flashing news at you, or some thing (your phone perhaps) in your hand to fidget with.

8. Just stop. And sit.

In addition to the practice of rest and respecting your ultradian rhythms, adopting an inner attitude of slowing down also goes a long way. No one else needs to notice. To whatever extent you push yourself to do more, do your best, and get as much done as possible, you can give yourself permission to do less, do a sufficient job, and not have to be perfect. You can turn more of your attention inward, to your connection to your baby and your body, even as you go about your work. No one owns your inner world, so smile at the idea of slacking off just a little bit. Be a little bit lazy. Trust me, if you are anything like the women I work with, your lazy will probably still be stellar, and you will enjoy life a bit more.

STOP WITH ME

Stop. Stop working. Stop trying to stop working.
Stop trying. Stop being lazy. Stop searching for meaning.
Stop landing anywhere. Stop acting confused. Stop.
Stop locking up your mysteries. Let me in. Stop rearranging
the surface features of your life. Stop thinking deep is deep. Stop thinking
blood is red. Stop hoarding the blood-red wisdom unborn in you.
There's got to be a better way. Do you love me? Stop loving
me. Stop unloving me. Stop tearing me apart.
Stop with me. Let's stop together. Six seconds. Ready. Set. Stop.
Now let's stop together forever,
and let the stopping go.
—BROOKE McNAMARA

LOOSENING YOUR GRIP

When the norm is short maternity leaves and superwoman expectations, and certainly not laziness and resting, it is difficult for many women to imagine deeply relaxing and receiving care for the first six weeks after giving birth.

The postpartum period is an invitation to sidle into a slower pace, which is why it is so useful to have had some practice experiencing stillness. One of the most remarkable facets of the postpartum experience—besides the miracle of having grown and birthed another human being—is the dramatic rhythm change in our lives. We are transported to a land where the pace is slow and languorous, and time has a hazy, mysterious quality. A day can pass so slowly that it seems it will never end. Yet weeks go by and it seems like we haven't changed our clothes, taken a shower, or done anything but laundry and nursing.

In these slow days, that voice inside you that judges your days by how much you have gotten done can get louder. Your self-image can be jarred when you have little to show for the day except sore nipples. We can mitigate this by adjusting our expectations. What would it be like to write a to-do list and then tear it up and throw it away? Try it! It sounds kind of funny, but letting go of expectations of productivity as a measure of success is a very real experience of a postpartum day when you have high hopes and nothing gets done, even though you feel you've been occupied during all of it.

JOURNALING YOUR INNER VOICES

Get out a piece of paper or a journal. If you are journaling about your pregnancy or just like to journal, you can certainly do this exercise in there, or you can buy a separate notebook or the like to do exercises in if you want to keep them separate.

- Begin by observing the voice that enters your mind, telling you that you should be doing more. What does it sound like? Who does it remind you of? What does it want from you? Give it full voice and write for five minutes from its point of view.
- Give the voice a name (something like Pest or Tyrant). When you see the narrative of this part written out, it will not have so much power over you. You will not get seduced into thinking that this voice is the whole story. Often, this voice wants you to stay in your mind and out of deep feeling. The mind feels safe and in control, while the feelings or the physical experience feels unpredictable and scary.
- Thank that voice for speaking up, and then return to the present moment and take a few breaths.
- Now turn to an inner voice, a kind voice that knows that just being who you are is enough, that your inner worth does not depend on what you do. This voice may be a mother, a higher self, or a fairy godmother. You can name her too. She is the one who knows that everything is okay, just as it is.
- Write to yourself from her voice. What does she want you to know?

In the future, when you notice you are being particularly hard on yourself, return to this full exercise, read what you wrote today to help you remember the difference between those two voices, or take a shortcut: Notice when the inner critic is running your mental show. Then simply pause and return to your breath. (No use arguing with this voice, because that is just giving it more attention.) Skip to the kind, encouraging voice. Call her by name if she has one. Choose a couple key phrases from that voice, like "everything is going to be okay" or "it's safe to rest," that soothe you, and repeat them slowly, feeling them reverberate through your body.

Habits of perfectionism and control can rear their heads during this time. Becoming a mother is a profound identity shift that will have your ego struggling to hold on. If we can practice yielding to, instead of fighting, some of the changes and be truly aware of the impermanent nature of all things, this time can be full of insights and spiritual ripening.

You have to be ready and willing to loosen your grip on who you are, so you can fully immerse yourself in the process of becoming who you will be. This change, however revelatory or dark, promises to be one of the most compelling and distinct transformations of your entire life. Having a baby strips you of your usual defenses, gives you an opportunity to act in new ways and see the world differently. There is the potential for deep insight into your self and the world around you. There is no going back to life as it was. So many things are going to change.

And yet, there is one thing that doesn't change—your inherent worth as a human being. Your value doesn't depend on how much you do or how much you give. It can be difficult to undo our programming regarding what makes someone "useful," but it is possible. Now is a great time to start. Being you is enough. Birthing, caring for, and feeding a growing baby and yourself as a new mother is enough.

LEAN INTO THE FEMININE

Growing up with a legacy of feminism, we have been encouraged to believe that we can do anything men can do—and maybe we can even do it better. We have penetrated institutions that were formerly exclusively male and not seen as women's domains. In the last fifty years, we have gained access to politics and the corporate world. There are more women than men pursuing higher education. In many ways, our striving has paid off. The gender gap is closing. A woman ran for president!

Yet there is one gender gap that can never close: at least for now, having a baby is something that only a female body can do. There is no experience that emphasizes the stark difference between female and male experiences like birthing and early parenting. However nontraditional our roles may have been with partners before, having a baby places different demands on a woman than it does on a man. Most women certainly recognize that intellectually, but the lived experience of this inequality can still be disarming for many women.

Here's the rub. Our grandmothers and mothers would have expected nothing less. Of course, as women, they would be more attuned to their babies and have to do more to care for them than their male counterparts. But younger generations of women have been raised with the possibility of egalitarianism in everything.

Community Stories:
Deena

Deena's anxiety postpartum was punctuated by how different her postpartum experience was from her husband's. She resented that only she could nurse, that she was expected to take the baby to the doctor and then report back on what happened, and that she was a virtual translator for her baby's needs. Even though it was she who was at home caring for the baby, she couldn't believe that, when her husband came home, she had to direct him on how to dress the baby and where to find diapers. She begrudged her deeper level of attunement to her baby. She could not believe how much bigger the demand was on her than her husband. For Deena, this seemed neither fair nor desirable. It took time for her to see the gifts in being able to feel so much closeness and synergy with her son.

When it comes to the postpartum period, this can be a big obstacle. Women have gone through all the physical changes of pregnancy and birth. While their partners have most likely accompanied these changes and have undergone their own shifts, it is the mother whose body has held and birthed the baby and is capable of feeding it. The mother-baby connection is a symbiotic relationship. It is not as simple as replacing those functions, like having the partner bottle feed with pumped breast milk. For the survival of the species, mothers are specially equipped to feel, understand, and respond to their babies' needs.

In addition to gender roles, there are the related principles of masculine and feminine that also get put under heavy renegotiation after having a baby. For centuries, healing systems have been looking through a dualistic lens of the universe. The Taoists have yin and yang. The yogis have Shakti and Shiva. In the West, we have feminine and masculine. Although people are starting to advocate for a nonbinary lens through which to see life, and non-dualism is a popular spiritual perspective in yoga, Buddhism, and Tantra, when it comes to birth, the principles of feminine and masculine are still very useful.

In order to succeed, many women have adopted qualities that are described as "masculine." Our culture values masculine qualities— like striving, rationality, and being competitive, independent, and steady—so we get reinforcement for adopting them. Making lists of goals, step-by-step projections of how to get there, and doing everything in your power to reach the destination are all masculine ways of moving through the world.

You might be thinking, *Well, how else do you get anything done?* There is certainly nothing wrong with these qualities when they are in balance. The challenge is that if you have been primarily operating with this masculine orientation, the postpartum period can be an unexpected and startling immersion into the world of the feminine.

To gracefully traverse this portal, the feminine strengths of inter-dependence, emotional attunement, and flexibility are paramount. Nestling up to the feminine may be as clear-cut as beginning to ask for help, softening the armor, releasing the need to do it all, and practicing graciously receiving. Embracing motherhood includes asking for help for things that you *could* do, but it doesn't have to be you doing them. Starting anything is always the hardest part. So practice flexing the muscle of asking for help and receiving it now, so that it will be stronger later.

Here are a few ways to start:

- Ask a simple favor of a friend or relative. For example, ask if you can come over for dinner or they can pick up takeout. Ask if they can do your laundry or come feed your animals. Ask if they can give you a foot massage. Ask someone to bring you a bouquet of flowers. Ask for something you might not normally ask for and that isn't a total necessity.
- When you receive a favor, resist the urge to reciprocate right away. Express your genuine appreciation and leave it at that.
- Cultivate a kind inner voice that reminds you that you don't have to do more. This could be in the form of the mantra "I have enough. I do enough. I am enough."
- When you hear the inner voice that insists that you can't stop until you have finished everything on your to-do list, return to your mantra. Train your mind to be satisfied and content with what you have done, rather than scanning for what you have not done.

SUMMARY

- The postpartum time is a rhythm shift, so understanding the need to rest and learning how to rest are crucial.
- Adjusting expectations, softening perfectionism, and taming your inner critic will set you up to enjoy the slow postpartum time.
- Our culture overvalues the masculine qualities of rationality, productivity, and independence. The postpartum period is a feminine time when emotional attunement, receptivity, and interdependence are key.

Practices

- Practice sitting and just being for five minutes. Don't check electronics, engage with anyone, or worry about meditation. Just sit and enjoy resting (and connecting with nature by sitting outside if possible).
- Respect your ultradian rhythms. After working or being active for ninety minutes, rest for ten minutes.
- Ask a friend for a meal, flowers, or a massage.
- Don't reciprocate a favor with a favor. Express your gratitude simply. (You don't need to write a thank-you note.)

Reflections

- What is your relationship to rest? What makes it easier for you to rest?
- When you feel stressed out or off-center, how do you get back on track?
- Make a list of free associations with the word "feminine."
- What do you anticipate might be difficult for you about the postpartum period? How is it for you to have unstructured time without a to-do list?

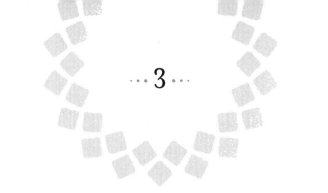

creating a postpartum
sanctuary plan

Planning for birth is both daunting and exciting. Women, couples, and health-care professionals usually cooperate and carefully consider what they want out of the birth experience. But our society would be a different place if there were as much attention given to the post-birth transition as there is to the birth itself. I venture to say that fewer women would be depressed, more couples would survive the first year, and babies would be calmer.

Just as your birth plan allows you to think through and communicate your ideal birth, a postpartum sanctuary plan is an excellent way to anticipate and plan for the support you will need to have the smoothest sacred window possible. I recommend that you create your plan with your partner in your third trimester. But before I guide you in putting together your postpartum sanctuary plan, there are a few things I want you to know.

First of all, you are going to need a lot more help than you think you will need. We tend to think that if we *can* do something ourselves, then we *should*. This is absolutely *not* true postpartum. All of your energy needs to go toward healing your body and learning about your baby. Just as you are providing unlimited food for your baby, you need someone to be nourishing you. And as tempting as it is, relying on partners for this care isn't the optimal setup for success, as they are going through their own journey into parenting.

Second, the purpose of receiving support at this time is not to help your baby—it is to help you. It is to support *you* in getting your basic needs of food, comfort, and unconditional love met, and also to support you in deepening your self-confidence and trusting in your instincts as a mother.

You will go through a range of emotions that you have never experienced, sometimes all in one day.

You will experience periods of doubt. You will need companionship that you can rely on, assuring you that everything is okay, that you will reemerge. You need someone who can reflect the richness of the process to you.

Having the support you need will allow you to immerse yourself in the experience as it is happening, so when it is time to surface, you will be completely intact. I have never heard a woman lament having too much postpartum support. I have only heard women regret that no one told them they should have invested more resources in postpartum care.

BUILDING YOUR POSTPARTUM SANCTUARY PLAN

Start with this question: What would it be like to set yourself up to have everything you need, and maybe even spoil yourself, during the sacred window? What would it be like to feel like a queen, to have your favorite healthy meals cooked and served to you, to have someone else doing the laundry and straightening up the house, to have a massage every week, physical therapy, and dreamy sleeps throughout the day with your best girlfriends and relatives around whenever you need them?

Pause for a moment. Close your eyes, and notice what that idea feels like in your body. Some women may experience a joyful, uplifting feeling. Others might feel discomfort because it seems indulgent or simply impossible to orchestrate. Yet others might feel dread at the thought of so much interaction and what feels like an invasion of privacy. Someone may experience a bit of all of them. Pay attention to your inner reaction: it has wisdom for you. Although for most of us receiving this kind of help seems like a luxury, postpartum, it is a necessity.

The postpartum sanctuary plan (see appendices 1 and 2) guides you through inquiries and information gathering that ensures you have all of the information and resources collected ahead of time to meet the five universal postpartum needs of rest, nourishing food, loving touch, spiritual companionship, and contact with nature after your baby is born.

You will find the postpartum sanctuary plan in three parts in the appendix. Appendix 1 is for you to fill out on your own. Appendix 2A is for both you and your partner to fill out separately and then compare, so make two copies. Appendix 2B is for you and your partner to fill out together.

After you fill these out, put them in a place that is easy to see, so that you remember to use them! What follows is some deeper explanation of values and reasoning behind the sanctuary plan.

Creating a Sanctuary

After having a baby, you will want your home to feel like a refuge. You'll be spending a lot of time there, so it is important that it feels good to you and that the people and the energy they bring also feel good. Consider now: Who do you want to visit you in the first three days? In the first two weeks? In the first month? Discuss this with your partner so you are in agreement, and then he or she can honor your wishes.

Here are some things you may want to consider when thinking of who you want to visit and when.

Primed hormonally to protect your baby, you will be more sensitive than usual to energy and words. Things that wouldn't normally bother you may get under your skin. This sensitivity is actually great news, it means that your mothering instincts are awake and that you know what you and your baby need at this time. Minimizing visitors is a good idea during the extended rest period. This may seem confusing in light of how much support you need. People who come to contribute are different from people who come to sit on the couch and admire your baby. Fortunately, with a little guidance, we can help people come into our home sanctuary in a way that will be helpful and supportive to us. I have included a sign, appendix 4, that you can put on your front door that will help with this.

Although there are the universal needs, support looks different for each woman. Contemplate the questions: What makes *you* feel supported and calm? Is it a straightened-up house? Is it a beautiful home-cooked meal? Is it a hug? A massage? Is it time to read a chapter of a book? Is it a bath drawn for you? A conversation with a friend?

When you know the answers, it is easier to ask for what you need.

A special note is required here for managing technology. Most of us are already well aware of the challenges of technology—the onslaught of text messages, e-mails, incoming calls, and the time suck and allure of Facebook, Instagram, Twitter, and Pinterest. This is a great time to reflect on how you want technology to work for you. Many of us are accustomed to browsing Google or playing games on our phones or scrolling through messages when what we actually need is downtime. Screen time complicates sleep patterns and often doesn't give us the mental break that we are looking for. Decide now what the optimal relationship to your phone, computer, and social media would be for you postpartum.

Would you like to look at your phone three times a day, in the morning, midday, and in the evening? Would you like to check e-mails once a day? Whatever you choose, you can let the people you are communicating with know so they know what to expect from you. This is huge in protecting your undistracted bonding time with your baby, as well as facilitating your own ability to rest.

Research shows that having a cell phone in sight changes the tone and topic of conversations, affecting our willingness to go deep and to concentrate. Better to keep your phone out of reach or, better yet, out of the room that you are resting or sleeping in, so you can concentrate on your baby and both of you can sleep soundly. Also, you will then be choosing when you want to use your phone or iPad, rather than picking it up mindlessly out of habit.

New moms are often tempted to use the Internet to research questions and clarify doubts. As you know, it is easy to fall into the online pit, spending more time than intended or becoming completely overwhelmed by the amount of information to sift through. Now is a good time to return to the old-fashioned way of gathering information about mothering: Talk to trusted mothers, grandmothers, friends, and health-care providers. Be courageous and reach out. Don't be afraid to use the words: "I am _____ (confused, afraid, in pain). This is what's happening. What do you think?"

Nourishing Your Body

Making sure you are well fed is one of the priorities of this postpartum period, and a great way to build and lean on community at this time.

One of the easiest places to start is with a meal train. It's great when the organizer of your baby shower or mother blessing is willing to organize the meal train. A baby shower is a gathering where people offer gifts for the baby. (A mother blessing is a ritual that honors the passage of the pregnant woman into motherhood. At a mother blessing, women gather together to share stories and lessons about birth and motherhood, making a piece of art together and creating a ritual for the new mom to gather strength for birth and motherhood.) If you don't have anyone to organize the meal train, go ahead and begin one yourself. It's worth it! There are free apps and websites, so you don't have to do all the asking and scheduling: www.mealtrain.com, www.mealbaby.com, and www.takethemameal .com are just a few options.

Start by brainstorming who in your family, neighborhood, or community may be able to help you. Women are often pleasantly surprised at the people who participate whom they would not necessarily have considered part of their support system. If you want to minimize the number of new people coming in and out of the house, you can have a basket or cooler outside your front door where people leave the meals. If you have specific food needs, state them. It's also great to give examples of your favorite meals, so people know what you like. Appendix 3 is a letter template for meal-train participants that you can use or modify.

In addition to a meal train, which usually lasts four to six weeks, set yourself up for success for the whole fourth trimester and beyond. Make a sample grocery list of the foods you like. Again, I have included some examples in appendix 5. With a list, someone else can easily shop for you. Also gather takeout menus, information for delivery services, and a list of restaurants that deliver. There's no quicker way to a meltdown than being hungry and tired while nursing your baby.

Gathering Your Tribe

A meal train is a great way to mobilize friends and neighbors who want to help you after you have a baby. The postpartum period is an amazing time to gather the people who want to support you, and mobilizing a meal train is a great start. For many people, having a baby is the beginning of building their tribe. Babies bring people together like nothing else. This is a chance to build a community to start supporting you now, one that can accompany you on this journey. The bonds that you form with other young parents, who you may not have had much in common with before, can evolve into rich and rewarding connections now that you have common questions and needs arising through parenting. These new connections are often one of the most memorable and nourishing parts of this phase of life.

It's also a great time to assemble a wider tribe or network of care providers. Likely, you have already started this process, but there may be resources in appendix 1 that you haven't considered, like lactation support, postpartum doula services, or a night nurse. It's best to get these recommendations now, so there is one less step to go through when you feel stressed or overwhelmed. The best place to find these resources is your friend network. If you are new to an area or the first of your friends to have a baby, venues where there is lactation support, birth centers, or midwifery collectives often have extensive references and contacts for postpartum services.

Remembering What Brings You Joy

Now that you know your body will be nourished, how will your mind and spirit be nourished? When you feel a little off, what gets you back on track? Here are some ideas to get you started:

Turning attention to your breath
Singing
Music
Movement
Reading inspirational words
Watching great films
Talking with a dear friend

Make a list of your own resources so you can visit it when things get rough. Be specific. If inspirational words soothe you, download podcasts or dharma talks so you have them readily accessible. Make a list of uplifting shows, films, or documentaries that you would like to watch. Have reading material available that is not on your phone or computer so that you are not dependent on, and then possibly distracted by, other features of your technology.

These small course corrections can make a big difference. When you start to get overwhelmed, you can pause, visit your list, and figure out which way sounds best to get the connection you need at that time. Place your list on your refrigerator or bathroom mirror, someplace that will remind you to check in and take a small action.

Safeguarding Your Relationship Postpartum

It's no secret that having a baby can create waves in relationships. Even when things go smoothly, a new baby brings an element of unpredictability that is a stressor on every couple. While becoming parents affects us in ways we could never imagine, there are some universal obstacles that we face. Dr. John Gottman, a seminal researcher on parenting and relationships, found that on average there is a 67 percent decline in marital satisfaction in the first three years after having a baby.

Community Stories:
Joanie

Joanie came to see me for a birth rehearsal, a process that I take pregnant women through in their last couple of weeks before birth so that they feel some of the sensations they will experience during birth ahead of time, as well as have access to pushing muscles before actually having to use them. The moment she stepped into my office, she was bereft. Her face was bright red and she was shaking, on the verge of tears. She felt pressured by both her mother and her mother-in-law to have them present at the birth and after. Even though she had moved thousands of miles away from both of them to avoid their interference, she felt guilty and confused about what to do. She felt consumed by their desires and unsure of what her responsibility was. She was absolutely sure that she wanted her birth experience to be between her, her baby, and her husband. She didn't want to have to fight to do things her way, but she was starting to realize that if she continued to be nice and agreeable, she would not have the experience she wanted.

The first session we worked through these old feelings of having to take care of other people. Her deep intuition was rearing up, encouraging her to unplug this legacy of caretaking from her own mother and mother-in-law, so she could redirect it to her baby and her new family. Like many women, she had a detailed birth plan and was preparing her body, mind, and spirit to have the birth she wanted. But when I asked about who would take care of her after the baby was born, if she didn't want her mother and mother-in-law there, Joanie drew a blank. She hadn't given it much thought, but imagined she would just figure it out with her husband. When I suggested to her that she would need to be nurtured and mothered as she became a mother, she cringed. She said that she hated the word *mothering* and had always been able to do everything herself.

I wish I could say that Joanie was the exception in thinking that her self-sufficiency, willpower, and resourcefulness would carry her through the postpartum period, but I hear this all the time. Together we talked about the five universal needs of postpartum women, and we came up with a plan of how she and her husband could be supported so she felt protected and safe while going through the uncertainty of learning about her new baby. We agreed that if she didn't receive any nurturing she might become even more resentful toward her own mother for not being able to give her that support. Instead, Joanie decided that a postpartum doula who would deliver nourishing food, walk her dog, and talk when she wanted to would be the most helpful. She wrote to me later to tell me that it was the best decision she ever made. She couldn't fathom the idea of having another baby without having this wise postpartum doula to support her.

The good news is that the research showed that, by addressing these obstacles ahead of time, it was possible to lower relationship distress as well as postpartum depression. Anticipating some potential roadblocks in your relationship goes a long way toward easing the transition to parenthood and even saving relationships. Specifically, Gottman's research found that all it took to mitigate the stress of the baby's first year on a marriage was two forty-minute counseling sessions before pregnancy to troubleshoot potential disagreements and prepare for what was to come. In appendix 2A, there are questions to use as starting points for these conversations, in case you don't make it to counseling. What follows are a context for those conversations and a few other suggestions for ways to deepen your relationship.

How to Approach Your Partner

While counseling sessions can be effective, you can also do some work on your own. The two of you are in this together, and there is no one in the world more invested in how you are doing than your partner. When you understand and acknowledge how interconnected your well-being is with your partner's well-being, it becomes obvious that what you are doing to your partner is what you are doing to yourself. In this way, your partner and your relationship can be your biggest allies and biggest untapped resources. Rather than just another thing that's demanding your energy, your relationship can become the power source for all the other areas of your life, the place you come back to in order to recharge and gain strength. This renewed understanding begins with unconditional positive regard, giving your partner the benefit of the doubt and acting with friendliness and kindness toward him or her. Stan Tatkin, the relationship expert and author of *Wired for Love*, says that, as couples, we need to form a relationship bubble. Inside that bubble are all the qualities that we stand for in our relationship, as well as what is sacred and private to us, and we need to protect this bubble.

A couple is made up of two individual people. The relationship is a third entity that has its own qualities and its own purpose. You may already have a strong sense of what your purpose is as a couple and for one another or you may still be discovering it. Perhaps having a child is part of your relationship's purpose. Reflecting on the beautiful qualities of your unique bubble will help the two of you to feel connected now, and give you something to refer back to.

THE COUPLE BUBBLE

1. Sit down together, each with a journal or piece of paper and pen. Set a timer for ten minutes and free-associate completing the following statements:

   • What I bring to us is . . .
   • What you bring to us is . . .
   • What we bring to the world, and what we have for each other is . . .
   • What we already are is . . .
   • Our compass or guiding principle is . . .
   • What I am committed to for me is . . .
   • What I am committed to for you is . . .
   • The wounds that I am healing include . . .
   • The wounds that you are healing include . . .
   • Our dreams are . . .

2. After ten minutes, share your answers with each other.
3. Take another sheet of paper and draw a Venn diagram—two circles that overlap in the middle. Make sure there is a big overlap in the middle. Label one circle with your name, the other with your partner's name. Label the middle "Us."
4. Fill in the circles together, choosing from the reflections you shared with each other. Create a visual representation that reminds you of what you are to each other and what the qualities and compass of your relationship are.

If you have made a formal commitment to each other, you may even want to revisit your vows or promises to one another and actually state them aloud. After all, the whole purpose of this exercise is to be very clear about your conviction to stay connected as a couple, as two become three.

VOWS

....

- Create a sacred space, go out into nature, or go to your favorite romantic restaurant. (Choose something that is in alignment with your relationship and connection.)
- If you have vows or promises that are important to you, bring them with you and say them aloud to each other.
- If you don't have any formal vows, reflect on these questions and share your answers with each other:

    What are three things that I appreciate about you as a partner?

    What do I commit to in our relationship after we become parents?

- Record your answers in a simple way, either making a voice recording or writing them down.

To fully show up in the relationship, to the "us," each of you has personal needs that must be met first. You reflected on your personal needs in the exercise above, now share those insights with your partner. Then ask your partner to reflect on his or her basic needs.

If your partner needs alone time, instead of both of you assuming that he can never have it again, brainstorm about how you might build that into a weekly routine. Would he rather have an hour every day or a half-day on the weekend? Does he need time to take a shower and sit down when he comes home from work in order to make the transition to home, or does he want to jump right in? Who could step in to be a primary support while he is gone? If an important part of your relationship has been the sexual connection, together think through how you will maintain intimate contact without penetration.

You probably already have a good idea of how your partner handles stress, but it is worthwhile to talk together about what your tendencies are when you are stressed. Here are some questions you should both answer about how you react to stress:

Do you withdraw?

Do you leave?

Do you talk a lot?

Do you get irritable?

When you notice how you are feeling, what is helpful for you?

What can your partner do to help you to get back on track?

What are you scared of?

What are the things that worry you about your relationship and how it will change as parents?

Are you afraid to lose a physically intimate connection?

Are you afraid of disappointing your partner?

Is it hard for you to be perceived as dependent or needy?

Are you afraid that you will become less important to your partner?

These questions, just like the personal needs you discussed before, will be used to help fill out your postpartum sanctuary plan.

If you have never explored the five love languages, finding out the way that your partner best receives support can be a revelation. The way that we show our love is not always the way our partner best receives it. It's our job to deliver the love, care, and compassion that can be received by our partner. You can take a test to see for yourself what your love language is at this website: www.5lovelanguages.com.

The five ways that we exchange appreciation are: touch, acts of service, words of affirmation, gifts, and quality time. You may already have an inkling which one of those lights you up the most, and which one your partner is most drawn to, but it's worth it to confirm your hunch. Remember that connecting through your love language is a way to express appreciation and communicate anything that may not be working for you.

There's a lot of research out there showing how stressful having a baby is on a relationship. If you listen to most people talking about it, it sounds like you are never going to have sex or an uninterrupted conversation again. But the good news is that there is also a lot of research showing that simple troubleshooting goes a long way toward strengthening your relationship long-term. Having a baby has the potential to bring you closer together rather than driving you further apart.

Ways to Stay Connected after Baby

Be learners together. Remember there is no right way to be a parent.

Express appreciation often.

Make time for honest conversations.

Remember your partner's love language and do the little things.

Allow your partner to find his or her own way with the baby.

Greet each other in comings and goings, when leaving the house and arriving.

Connect before sleep and upon waking, with eye contact or a verbal greeting.

Dedicate three to five minutes a day for loving connection, whether that is gazing into each other's eyes, light touch, or talking.

SUMMARY: PREPARING FOR YOUR POSTPARTUM SANCTUARY PLAN

- A postpartum sanctuary plan is just as important as a birth plan in setting yourself up for success in the fourth trimester.
- Plan to need a lot of help and be creative about where you might get it. Build your tribe.
- Assemble your network of health care providers and therapists now so that it is there if and when you need it.
- Many relationships suffer after having children, but if you make the health of your relationship a priority, your partnership can thrive.

Practices

- Makes copies of the postpartum sanctuary plans, appendices 1 and 2. Discuss them with your partner. Fill them out and stick them somewhere where you will see them and use them.
- Gather takeout menus, information for delivery services, and a list of restaurants that deliver, assembling the information that you need.
- Discover the unique qualities of your couple bubble.
- Review your vows and promises to one another, or create some.
- Find out what your love language is as well as that of your partner. Taking into account your partner's love language, do something to surprise him or her.

Reflections

- How can you start to build the sanctuary you want to heal in?
- Who is in your life that you can turn to for specific things, and what sources do you still need to track down?
- What do you appreciate most about your partner and your partnership?
- What agreements would you like to make with your partner?
- What is one thing that you could start doing now that you would like to continue after your baby is born?

··· 4 ···

third trimester:
preparing your body for birth

Birth is more than just a physical event—it is a mental, sexual, spiritual, whole-being experience. Intuitively, most women know this. That's why it feels daunting. We know that getting all the right information, being in great shape, and having a supportive team are important preparatory elements. We also know that even with the best preparation possible, it will still be a walk through the fire.

If all we knew of pregnancy and motherhood were the images online and in magazines, we might conclude that it is a weight-gain and weight-loss challenge, rather than the powerful rite of passage and total transformation that it is. We are seduced by the idea of upholding the superwoman myth; we see pregnant women and new mothers doing it all, even at the gym and in the yoga studio. Resting and slowing down are hard to show on an Instagram account, but doing a handstand on a cliff at forty weeks pregnant draws a lot of attention and awe.

In many ways, we are rewarded for looking invincible and unstoppable—but it doesn't benefit our own long-term peace and sanity. Our families and our jobs may really like this superhuman stamina, but most of all, our egos like it. In fact, it's mostly our egos that won't let us off the hook.

As women, we receive all kinds of mixed messages about how much exercise we should do and what kinds of exercise are safe during pregnancy. Ultimately, it would be great if we could just tune in and listen to our bodies. However, when so much is changing so quickly, it is sometimes hard to know what our bodies are saying and what really is good for us. When should we push ourselves? When should we rest? What will facilitate more ease both short-term and long-term, and what is just falling into habits? The truth is that what might feel good right now might not be what is beneficial long-term.

EXERCISE JUST ENOUGH

A key to preparing for birth is, indeed, being active. We all lie somewhere on the spectrum from very active to not active at all, and pregnancy is a time to move toward balance. Doctors are famous for telling pregnant women, "Just keep doing what you're doing, but don't start anything new." For the most part, this is wise advice: women can continue doing the physical exercise that they have always loved with some slight modifications. But this doesn't hold true for everything. If you work at a desk and don't like to exercise much, you'll want to start moving more. Movement is just the right medicine for the aches and pains of a growing pregnant body. Gentle exercise, like walking, swimming, or prenatal yoga, are critical to your circulation, your overall body awareness, and a sense of self-confidence that your body is reliable, strong, and supple.

As stated earlier, birth is much more than a physical experience, but you will want to feel connected to your body, to know that it is trustworthy and capable. Connection to your body and a positive birth experience are key ingredients to feeling good, and sane, postpartum. Many women use pregnancy as a motivator to get in shape, while some very active women may be reluctant to—but need to— slow down as they move through their pregnancies.

Many of the women with whom I work are extremely active. Their criteria for being in shape rival that of an amateur athlete. They are in formidable shape, and exercising regularly is a foundational part of their lives. When I ask them about their postpartum plan and what they have identified as resources for when they are feeling stressed, they almost all say yoga, Pilates, or running. Of course, these are healthy options; exercise is a healthy stress reliever, but sometimes it is the only way that women know how to regulate their stress levels. Pregnancy is a time to soften the grip on high-impact activities and heavy lifting, so it is a great time to strengthen internal practices like meditation, so that you don't require such high levels of exercise in order to get through the week. The idea here is to back off, to learn to rest, and to get more out of less. This will serve you well in the postpartum period when you cannot exercise safely with such rigor.

I get concerned when I meet women who are rigid about shifting their routines, women who say, "I absolutely will not stop riding my bike. And if I find a doctor who asks me to, I won't work with her." Or, "My body is feeling great at CrossFit. There's no reason to stop." Why is it so hard for us to let go? And then I remember how everywhere we look, we are inundated by images of women's bodies. While in past generations women dressed to hide their bellies, today women wear formfitting dresses to accentuate their pregnant shapes. Articles get widely shared on social media with some version of how incredible it is that a pregnant woman is still doing a particular activity.

Recently, a fitness company that specializes in prenatal and postpartum fitness released a new logo that is a woman with a big pregnant belly holding a huge barbell over her head. Another popular picture on the social-media fitness pages is a ballerina in pointe shoes doing a flawless arabesque, clearly near or at nine months pregnant. Yoga practitioners regularly post pictures of themselves doing handstands and headstands with a big belly. The message is, *Just because I'm pregnant, it doesn't mean I have to stop what I am doing.*

I am a superwoman, and the fact that I can still perform as if I were not pregnant proves how unstoppable I am.

These pictures generate huge amounts of attention and enthusiasm. They are ego boosters; friends and strangers chime in to cheer the women on in these amazing feats. We live in a culture that glorifies overdoing, and pregnancy is no exception.

But the truth is, deciding what to do and how to do it while pregnant is more complicated than at other times. It's important to know that your pregnant body is a changing body and *how* it is changing. There are different strains and demands on it than there are normally. Your body is producing a hormone called *relaxin* that softens ligaments and joints. Its function is to help the joints of the pelvis open to make space for the baby to pass through. However, relaxin doesn't just work on the pelvis. It affects all the joints in the body. Joints become looser and less stable. With joints that are less stable, the weight of the body is more difficult to support.

Compressive exercise, like running and weightlifting, places even more strain on an already unstable foundation. In response, muscles often get tighter to try to provide the support that the ligaments no longer can. When the muscles of the pelvic floor tighten and shorten, birthing a baby becomes more complicated and can contribute to pelvic-floor dysfunction down the line. Even with great form and correct posture, the amount of downward pressure on the pelvic floor that is placed by the weight of the baby together with additional weight or bouncing is often too much for the pelvic floor to withstand.

The challenge for women is that the consequences of overexerting are often not immediate, so we feel like we are listening to our bodies and are then caught by surprise when birth or postpartum recovery, or even menopause, are difficult. We need to develop a long-term view of our health, taking care of our life force and changing bodies so we can use them how we want into old age.

When joints and ligaments are loose, stretching can become easier.

Yoga practitioners are often pleased when they are pregnant and can stretch much farther than they could before. What many women don't realize, because it is hard to feel, is that the added stretch they are gaining is not because the muscles are more flexible but because their ligaments are overstretching. Ligaments are like strong rubber bands, taut and difficult to stretch. However, once stretched, they don't resume their original shape easily. Overstretching ligaments while pregnant often contributes to lower back and sacroiliac joint pain, as well as prolapse, postpartum.

A study done by PLOS ONE of 1,500 mothers found that 77 percent experienced persistent lower back pain over a year after giving birth, and 49 percent experienced urinary incontinence. And a study published in the *American Journal of Obstetrics and Gynecology* found similar degrees of lasting pelvic pain in women who had cesarean sections compared to those who gave birth vaginally, which could indicate the pain is due to the time leading up to giving birth, as opposed to the birth itself.

You do not need to be afraid to move. Your pregnant body will benefit from everyday activities like walking, gardening on all fours, and squatting, rather than what we typically default to, which is alternating between sitting and high-impact exercise. If you are a runner, an athlete, or an elite yoga practitioner, the real challenge is not to maintain everything you have been doing. While to the outside eye, the high mileage and intricate inversions are impressive, if you are honest, you probably know that it is psychologically harder for you to stop doing them than it is physically for you to continue doing them.

Remember that this is not a forever adjustment. Truly backing off for the last months of pregnancy and the first few months postpartum will mean that you can return to what you love intact and build to the intensity that you like sooner. This pause will set you up to be able to do what you love longer, without pain, and to have decent amounts of energy sooner after giving birth.

EXERCISES FOR PREPARING YOUR BODY FOR BIRTH AND EASING PREGNANCY PAIN

Below are some exercises that you will absolutely want to do on a regular basis as you get closer to giving birth. These are gentle exercises that take into account your looser joints, your changing body, your lower energy levels, and the ways you can prepare your body for giving birth.

Protect Your Lower Back and Practice Supportive Posture

At some point, every pregnant woman has caught a glimpse of her profile in a mirror or store window and been surprised. A pregnant body is constantly in flux, shifting to redefine its center of gravity. For the body to realign itself to support the new weight of growing breasts and a growing belly, not to mention the softer ligaments that are the base of support for the spine and torso, there is a lot going on!

It doesn't help that our lifestyles, with more sitting, texting, and computer work than ever, predispose us to the postural adaptations that pregnancy also leans toward.

To compensate for growing breasts, our shoulders begin to round and our heads jut forward. To compensate for the growing belly, many women tuck their tailbones, flattening their glutes and pushing the pelvis forward. Others succumb to the weight of the baby that pulls them into a swayback. All of these habits can create compression in the lower back (see fig. 1).

So what should you do? It starts with awareness. Notice if these postural tendencies are familiar. The truth is you are bringing your prepregnancy posture with you, and pregnancy will probably exaggerate your habits. Make a conscious choice to practice supportive posture. Whether your lower back is already a source of discomfort, or if it's just to support and keep your spine supple as your belly continues to grow, you will want to practice lengthening the muscles along your lower back. There are several ways to avoid that shortened feeling that causes pain in your lower back.

Awareness starts with breathing, something we are already doing all the time, though not always consciously. Ideally, these exercises are practiced with an exercise ball. An exercise ball is an inexpensive tool that requires us to be making micro adjustments with our internal balancing system, keeping our body more awake than sitting on the ground or a chair does. A ball is also a great tool for birthing and for bouncing on with a fussy baby. If you don't have a ball, you can still get great benefit from these exercises by sitting up—not slumping—in a chair.

Fig. 1: Postural profiles before pregnancy, during pregnancy, and postpartum

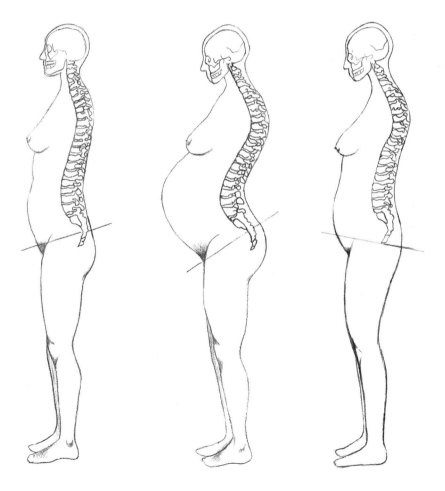

BREATH FOR LENGTH

....

Taking care of your lower back and maintaining great alignment begins with your breath. This particular breath is for everyone and touches on posture as well as pelvic-floor preparation. I call this the breath for length because it lengthens the curves of your spine.

1. As you focus on your inhalations, allow your ribs to expand first and then your belly to fill. You want to feel your whole trunk expand.

2. Your breath will extend all the way to your pelvic floor, explained in detail below, which you want to drop and spread. For now, you can just allow the exhale to happen. If you have been taught to breathe diaphragmatically, puffing your belly on inhalations, this will be a new approach. To inhale into your chest and ribs, you want to keep your abdominals engaged a bit, so your ribs can fill first. It is important that your ribs move, lift, and expand when you inhale, and it takes practice at first.

3. Place your hands on your side ribs, with your fingers facing each other, and feel your hands move away from each other on your inhale and back toward each other on your exhale, like an accordion (see fig. 2).

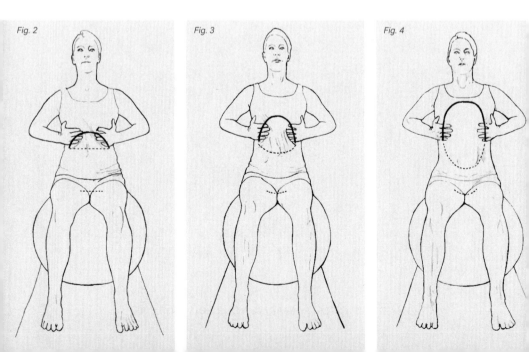

Fig. 2   Fig. 3   Fig. 4

4. On the exhale, maintain the lift in your ribs as you pull your belly toward your spine. Then at the end of your out breath, let your ribs relax and return to their original position (see fig 3).

5. On your next breath, when you exhale, coordinate the movement of your abdominals toward your spine with the lift of your pelvic floor. Engage your abdominals toward your spine and draw your pelvic floor in and up at the same time (see fig. 4).

Note: At first, it is really helpful to practice this sitting on the exercise ball if possible because it has a soft and responsive surface, making it easier to feel pelvic floor movement. On any surface, you can visualize your *pelvic diamond*—the area between your pubic bone, sitting bones, and tailbone (see fig 5). When you inhale, you want to feel your pelvic floor widening and opening to the surface of the ball, and then, as you exhale, feel the diamond shrinking and the pelvic muscles moving away from the ball.

There are many different ways to breathe, but the above breath will help you engage your core and will be an essential touchstone for your postpartum recovery.

Fig. 5: The pelvic diamond

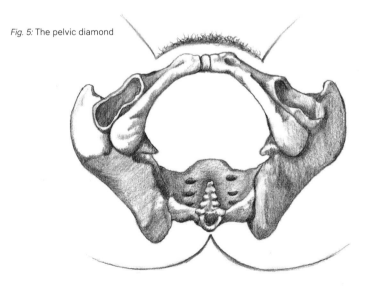

What Is the Pelvic Floor?

What exactly is the pelvic floor? It is a multitiered group of interweaving muscles that surround the lower openings of your body and also serve as a shelf for your reproductive and digestive organs. What does that mean? The first tier of muscles makes sure that sex and elimination are working optimally. The first tier of muscles is important for birth, because the baby's head stretches them considerably, and if they are too taut or don't have enough time to adjust, they may not soften enough and may tear when your baby emerges.

The second tier is important because those muscles make sure that your organs are in the right place, which is a pretty vague concept if they have always been in the right place. It is usually only when something goes wrong with organs that we really notice them, and then it's all we think about. When that second tier of muscles is strained or pulled, the organs start to slip below where they are meant to be, which causes sensations of heaviness and fullness.

CAT POSTURE

....

Coordinating simple movements with your breath can also provide welcome relief from lower back pain. Try the cat posture (see fig 6).

From all fours, as you exhale, press into the ground, hug your baby toward your spine, drop your head and round your back. Breathe freely into your back as you feel the long muscles of the spine widening. Then, allow your body to make gentle movements, shifting your hips and head from side to side as it feels good. Then, return to a neutral spine, and as you exhale again, round your back. Do this five times, really feeling your belly, your baby, and your back.

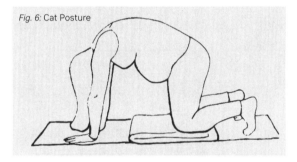

Fig. 6: Cat Posture

WALL SQUAT

....

Squat against a wall, with your thighs at a ninety-degree angle. Press your lower back, shoulders, and the back of your head against the wall. Place your hands on your belly and as you exhale, press your lower back to the wall and feel your hands move closer to each other. Hold the squat while breathing freely for thirty seconds. You may have to really scoop your tail forward to get your lower back against the wall—that's fine! This is great for keeping those muscles supple and relieving pain in them, but don't worry. You don't have to stand like that all the time. Normal standing posture allows for a gentle curve in your lower back. This exercise helps to release taut lower back muscles that will allow you to stand normally with more ease.

UPPER BACK STRETCH

....

The wall squat and cat posture both provide great immediate relief, but sometimes, discomfort can accumulate. When that happens, there are a few possible culprits. Your upper back may need to lift and open to make space for your lower back to lengthen and so that your diaphragm and pelvic floor have space to move.

To open your upper back, interlace your hands behind your head. Lean your head into your hands, inhale, and look up (see fig. 7). Include your entire upper back, not just your head, in the movement, moving all the way from the bottom of your ribs (without arching your lower back). You should feel more space opening between your baby and your ribs. When you exhale, drop your elbows forward and your chin toward your chest.

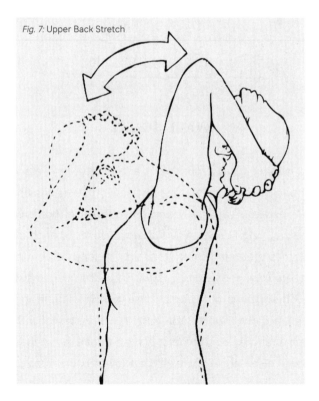

Fig. 7: Upper Back Stretch

Stabilize Your Pelvis

As well as the shortening of the lumbar curve, what also might be contributing to lower back discomfort is instability in your pelvic bones. Many prenatal yoga classes focus on hip openers during pregnancy. This can be very helpful for women who are just starting yoga. However, if you are a longtime yoga practitioner, I don't recommend hanging out in hip-opening postures like *baddhakonasana* and *upavista konasana*, relaxing into the even greater sense of opening that is available because your ligaments are becoming looser. As I mentioned above, when ligaments are overstretched it is hard for them to return to their normal length and strength.

This can lead to lower back and sacroiliac pain after giving birth, which takes a great deal of time to alleviate. If your pelvis feels unstable and you've got a lot more swagger than normal, you can wear a thin, soft belt, like a yoga strap, around your pelvic bones, at the level of your thighbones, to minimize wobbliness. Many women find it a great relief. If it feels good, I recommend wearing such a belt during yoga practice during the last trimester.

The attention that you place on how you hold yourself now, during pregnancy, will set you up to be able to breastfeed, baby-wear, and walk with comfort after you have your baby, so it is worth your devoted attention now!

Tone and Relax Your Pelvic Floor

"Do more Kegels!" That's the extent of advice and information that most women receive about their pelvic floors. Rarely are women assessed to find out if they actually need these exercises, taught how to do them correctly, or checked to see if they are doing them effectively. Learning how to find and use your pelvic floor muscles (see fig. 8) will be one of your biggest secret weapons in birth and postpartum. The more familiar you get with this territory, the more you will learn how to both engage and soften these muscles, and the easier it will be for you to find them again after having a baby.

Including your pelvic floor is the final piece to your lower back comfort. A proper pelvic-floor exercise will teach you how to pull up and in as well as push down and out. If you want a guided audio practice that leads you through the anatomy as well as guides you to a proper Kegel exercise, go to www.magamama.com/pelvic-mapping and download an audio guide.

Fig. 8: The pelvic floor muscles

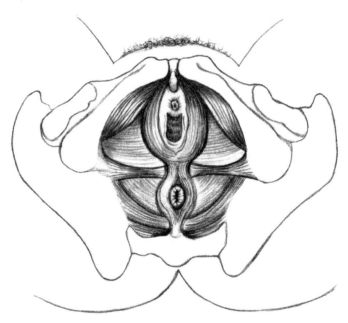

The Goldilocks principle applies as much to the pelvic floor as it does to exercise. I have had very few women—two to be exact—come to see me because they thought their pelvic floors were too tight. Almost every woman who comes to see me is sure that her pelvic floor is not strong enough. In fact, the cause of pelvic-floor dysfunction is split almost down the middle, evenly divided between women who could use more support and tone in their pelvic floor and women whose muscles need to let go and relax.

So how do you know where you stand on this spectrum? First, if you are a horseback rider, runner, yoga practitioner, or a Pilates or barre-method junkie, you most likely have a very strong and tight pelvic floor. Your work will be to learn to let go to create an easy exit for your baby and minimize tearing. While you can seek out a pelvic-floor physical therapist to help you prepare for birth—and you can also schedule a post-birth appointment with that professional—there is a lot that you can do on your own to prepare.

FULL-RANGE BREATHING

Again, it starts with the breath. We'll add a step to the breath for length. While it teaches you to soften your pelvic floor on the inhale and engage on the exhale, there is actually another phase that is crucial to pelvic health—bearing down.

Begin on the exercise ball, if you have one, with the breath for length, and then, on your next exhale, push your pelvic floor toward the ball. Since you are pregnant, and especially if you have a history of prolapse, you won't want to use your full strength to bear down, but you will want to find the muscles that work to do that. It will probably take some experimentation if you have only ever been pulling these muscles in and up.

Imagine a bodybuilder who does a lot of bicep curls. Her arms are probably permanently bent, even when she is relaxed. If you tell her to straighten her arm, she won't be able to do so without added weight or pressure. If you have done exercises where you squeeze your inner thighs a lot or activate *mula bandha* (which is Sanskrit for "root lock" and is practiced in yoga) your pelvic floor is the equivalent of that bent arm—it's constantly engaged. Pushing these muscles down, as if you were trying to expel a lover, will stretch them, making them more elastic. You will be using these muscles' full range of motion. In the last month of your pregnancy, you can let go of the contracting phase in the breath for length altogether. Just focus on relaxation and gentle pushing during the exhales.

BALL MASSAGE

Another way to soften these hard-to-reach muscles is by using tennis balls. The pressure will help tense muscles relax. Place a tennis ball on the outside of one sitting bone, gently and cautiously sitting on it. Then roll it around in a horseshoe shape, until it's on the other side of your sitting bone. Try it on both sides. Oftentimes an impediment to activation or release is simply contacting areas of rigidity or places with which you don't have easy proprioceptive awareness.

You can also experiment by placing the ball on your tailbone and then tracing your whole pelvic diamond with it. Spend time in the places that feel foreign or very painful, so you can allow time for the muscles to release and widen.

MASSAGE THE PERINEUM

You can also manually stretch your perineal muscles, but please note: if you have been told not to have sex during your pregnancy, then you will want to avoid perineal massage.

Stretching your own perineal muscles can be a little physically awkward with a big belly to contend with, but it's possible. Prop yourself up at a sixty-degree angle, open your legs, and use a little bit of lubricant on your thumbs. Place your thumbs on the inside of your vaginal opening, about an inch inside, and press straight down toward your tailbone. Hold them down for a minute or so, until you feel a stretch and maybe discomfort but not pain. Then begin moving your thumbs in a semicircle, pausing where there is tension, to encourage and allow the tissue to let go.

You can start at thirty-six weeks, and you will need to do this for at least ten minutes a day to feel a significant difference. Many women come to me for birth rehearsals, during which I do the perineal stretching for them. They usually relate that what I do is nothing like what they were doing by themselves or with their partners. Without knowing the territory in an anatomical way, most people are tentative about stretching the muscles in that area. You want to challenge the tissue and sustain that stretch without being aggressive; the stretch is what will allow for true birth preparation. A moderate level of discomfort is necessary for it to be effective. In my office, I work up to sliding a full fist inside, so that women can gain the confidence, both mentally and physically, that something the size of a baby's head will be able to fit without incredible pain. Studies are mixed on whether perineal massage is useful, but those results could be skewed because most people aren't taught how to do it properly.

If you are questioning whether you're doing the perineal massage right, it's worth it to schedule an appointment with a pelvic-floor physical therapist or a sexological bodyworker to teach you how to do it and practice with you. This is especially important for yoga teachers, ballet dancers, Pilates practitioners, barre-method enthusiasts, and horseback riders who have extremely strong and tight pelvic floors and are disproportionately disposed to pelvic-floor injuries during childbirth.

If you adequately prepare your pelvic floor, you are creating connection and confidence, are already in touch with this intimate part of your body, and are more likely to trust it when things get more intense. You are also setting yourself up for a shorter pushing stage, which means you are less likely to damage nerves and tissue. Coming through birth in one piece sets you up for a less painful, more joyful, and shorter postpartum recovery.

CROSS-TRAINING YOUR NERVOUS SYSTEM

Even more important than training our bodies for birth is training our nervous systems. Even if you have been walking, squatting, swimming, and visualizing softening and relaxing your pelvic floor, there is almost nothing that can convince this most vulnerable and intimate part of your body to open if you are feeling afraid or threatened. So getting to know yourself and how your physiology works under stress can be one of the most helpful tools you can have during birth. Start with this simple exercise—the one-minute game.

ONE-MINUTE GAME

1. Set a timer for sixty seconds and start it.
2. Imagine one of your favorite places in nature, where you have great memories. As you call forth that image, notice the sensations in your body. Notice how your breath feels. Is it slower or faster, more or less noticeable? Notice how your skin feels. Notice the muscles of your face. What about your pelvis?
3. Stay with that image for one minute and notice how you feel after that short experiment.
4. Next, restart your timer and imagine that you are in a hurry to get out the door in the morning and you can't find your car keys. You are looking all over for them. You're going to be late if you don't find them.
5. Now notice your breath and your heart rate. Compared to your Hawaiian beach or pine forest, it's probably pretty uncomfortable.
6. Stay with it and continue to notice what happens in your body. How does your skin feel? How about the muscles of your face, your jaw, and your pelvis?
7. After a minute of that, notice your overall state, your mood and emotions, as well as the physical sensations.

When you are in one of your favorite places in nature, it is pleasurable. You feel safe and protected, as though there is nothing to worry about. You don't have to think about relaxing; you just relax, because the environment is so soothing and comfortable. The conditions are there for you to relax, and so you do. Your breath and heart rate slow down. Your jaw relaxes, and your facial muscles might light up in a smile. Your skin feels soft and porous. On the other hand, when you are searching for your keys, it's stressful. Your heart is probably racing, your breath is faster or you may hold your breath altogether. Your jaw tightens; your brow furrows. You may feel aggravated, frustrated, or outright angry. At the end of the minute, you're probably dying to return to the earlier vacation!

The nervous system is responsible for initiating all of the impulses that become actions in the body. Everything from moving your arm to picking up a fork you dropped to sending the message to your bowels to release to regulating your body temperature. Your *sympathetic nervous system* is in charge of actions. It is responsible for the active phase of the ultradian rhythms. Remember earlier when we discussed how the natural cycles of your body have ninety minutes of action and movement and then ten minutes of rest? The sympathetic nervous system is dominant during the phase of action in the ultradian rhythm.

Your *parasympathetic nervous system* is in charge of the resting phase of the ultradian rhythms. The sympathetic and parasympathetic nervous systems work together, continually shifting their ratios of activation to create *homeostasis*, or balance. We need both functioning healthily to have all the energy we need to live the lives we want—and the capacity to rest is part of that.

Under duress, however, our nervous systems function differently. Your sympathetic nervous system is responsible for the fight-or-flight response. This response is designed to protect us from danger, to deal with a threatening situation swiftly either by fighting or getting away as fast as possible. Evolutionarily, it was functional to escape wild animals. But nowadays, for most of us, our fight-or-flight response is overreactive. Ongoing stresses like traffic, jam-packed schedules, and role juggling—stresses that are not actually life-threatening—register as such in the nervous system. This leads to depletion as the body secretes stress hormones like adrenaline and cortisol on an ongoing basis, constantly draining reserves that were designed for only occasional use.

You probably felt the sympathetic-nervous-system response in your body when you imagined hurriedly looking for your keys, as your heart rate increased and your focus narrowed. There are also emotions that correspond with the two branches of the nervous system. Depending on how great a threat is or is perceived to be, in addition to how frequently a person experiences this reaction, a person may experience irritation, frustration, anger, or even rage.

When responding to threat or danger, your parasympathetic nervous system also functions differently. Your body may freeze and become immobilized. You can recognize this as the look of a deer in headlights. When faced with something scary, we may become unable to speak or even move. We are stunned. This response is beyond the level of the rational mind. In this state, we can't force ourselves or be forced to move or talk. A more extreme response of the parasympathetic nervous system is total collapse. In animals, we call this "playing dead." In humans, this may look like losing control of our elimination functions or passing out. Emotionally you may experience apathy, resignation, fear, or helplessness.

Wild animals don't experience trauma, while humans and domesticated animals do. Rarely as humans do we allow ourselves—and are we allowed—the chance to go through the complete cycle of activation and deactivation. This process takes time, and in our fast-paced lives, we don't always take it.

Imagine that while walking down the street, you trip and fall down. Most of us feel embarrassed to fall down, which causes us to skip steps to an integrated recovery. We don't slow down to notice where or how we are. Without taking stock of whether or not we are hurt or how we are feeling, we pop right up and continue walking, eyes locked forward, so we don't have to make eye contact with anyone who might have seen us. Our social relationships and self-consciousness can alter our necessary biological responses, so we don't fully process an experience. Of course, tripping is a fairly mild example, but nonetheless these incomplete responses are cumulative.

The Wolf and the Rabbit

Trauma is a scary word that most of us want to avoid. Most of us either overidentify or under-identify with it. We think either "I'm totally traumatized" or "I don't have any trauma at all." The truth is that all of us have experienced trauma. I wish there were a better word for it that wasn't so daunting or stigmatizing. Trauma is simply part of being human. Fortunately, healing is also a hallmark of being human. The best way to understand trauma is to observe the behavior of wild animals. As you read the following story, I invite you to notice the sensations in your own body.

Imagine a wolf hunting a rabbit. The wolf, salivating and pacing, starts its careful approach, getting closer and closer. At some point the rabbit senses that it is being stalked and stops moving (freezes). If the wolf continues approaching, the rabbit will play dead (collapse). Then, if the wolf is still interested, it will come pick up the rabbit by the neck and shake it around to confirm if the rabbit is dead or not. Predators don't usually want dead prey. If the wolf is convinced the rabbit is dead, it will simply drop it and run off. When the rabbit senses that the wolf is gone, then it opens its eyes to look around (visual orientation), then its little ears perk up and flash back and forth (auditory orientation). Then, if, through its senses, the rabbit perceives that it's safe, the rabbit bolts upright, coming up to all fours, continuing to look around in the environment. Next the rabbit shakes, and continues shaking (discharge/deactivation) until a seemingly spontaneous ending when the shaking finishes and it runs off.

When one of the branches of the nervous system, sympathetic or parasympathetic, doesn't go through a complete cycle, from activation to deactivation, it creates a short circuit. When the system short circuits, it creates a groove or loop, a repeating pattern. Then, when we face a challenging or stressful situation, our system responds in the same way it did in past situations that our body perceives to be analogous. In the above situation of falling down, our social shame sends us into autopilot. Overriding the need to pause, slow down, and recover, we spring into action. If we imagine the frames of an old filmstrip, when we experience trauma, it is as if our mind skips some frames of the film. The body continues on, but there is incongruence between what the body experiences and what the mind records. This fragmented experience results in trauma and an inability to be in the present moment.

GAME OF THREES

Stress and trauma make it difficult to stay in the present moment. When we experience stress, our body and mind replay past memories or project future scenarios. A simple and important tool to help you attune to the present moment is the game of threes. You can do this anywhere, anytime.

1. From wherever you are—your bedroom, the doctor's office, your bathroom—look around you. Notice three things in the environment: for example, a family picture, a water glass, and a shirt.
2. From this same place, notice three things about yourself: for example, the skin on my face feels warm, I'm excited about this book, my belly is tight.
3. Pause between each object, sensation, or feeling that you have. Go back and forth between what you see outside yourself and what you perceive inside yourself three times.
4. Then notice how you feel overall. What happened as a result of this noticing?

This shift of attention from what's around you back to what is inside you will help you to stay in the present moment, and remain calm. You may need to actively work with your mind. When it starts making associations such as "family picture" . . . "my mom is driving me crazy" . . . "I hope she doesn't come to the hospital too early" . . . come back to the object itself. Let the family picture simply be a family picture. If that's impossible, then find another object that has less difficult associations. Choose the objects with ease, and with this pendulation between your outside world and inside world, allow yourself to be more comfortable and at ease in your own skin.

When it comes to giving birth, we are working with the most intimate parts of our bodies, which requires safety and protection. In the past, that may not have always been what our bodies received. An overwhelming number of women have experienced sexual assault. Others have had unpleasant gynecological exams and procedures, abortions, or miscarriages. When a baby comes through this territory, although it is a "normal" physiological event, birth doesn't always seem normal to the body. Birth has the potential to trigger one of our nervous-system loops. For example, it may provoke a freeze response in someone who has been sexually assaulted or had previous negative birth or gynecological experiences.

If you are a survivor of sexual assault, or have gone through a difficult journey with fertility, pregnancies, loss, or abuse, seek a counselor who can help you to restore your nervous system's responses so that you can show up fully empowered for the birth of your child. Somatic Experiencing trauma resolution therapy is a powerful modality that can help you free yourself from the residue of those previous patterns, and arrive at your birth with less carryover from earlier difficult experiences. Having a doula who knows your history at the birth can also be extremely helpful, so that you remain oriented, feel supported, and know what your options are if you start to feel confused or disoriented. People who have a history of hospital trauma might consider alternative birthing options like birth centers or home births, so as not to set in motion previous trauma loops. With awareness and support, we have the chance to avoid further trauma and even repair past trauma. We can have a restorative experience, where our nervous system demonstrates resilience and we emerge from birth more whole and more empowered. This is essential in setting ourselves up for success in the postpartum period.

IDENTIFYING YOUR NERVOUS SYSTEM'S RESPONSE

1. All day long, we respond to little stresses, and they are not always bad things. They are as simple as your phone ringing in the doctor's office, a friend saying an unkind word, a full e-mail box, or receiving a generous gift or an unexpected compliment. Close your eyes and imagine each one of those scenarios.

2. When you feel what it would be like for your phone to ring in a doctor's office, is your impulse to want to hide or run out? That's the flight response. Is your impulse to ignore it and wait until it's over? That's the freeze response. Is your impulse to get mad at whoever is calling and interrupting you? These might be split-second responses, but they are helpful at letting you know how your wiring works.

3. Also, imagine that you just had a delicious two-week vacation prior to these scenarios happening. Your reaction would probably have much less intensity.

4. On the other hand, if you had just had a very stressful week, maybe a fight with your partner, or a fender bender, and then one of these scenarios happened, your ability to attenuate your reactions would be much less.

Ina May Gaskin, midwife and pioneer of natural childbirth, is famous for saying, "Open mouth, open cervix." She is talking about relaxing the jaw to relax the pelvic floor, which allows the baby to come out, instead of clenching and resisting. Clenching the jaw and tensing muscles are sympathetic-nervous-system fight responses. Imagine a dog growling and defending its territory. On the other hand, the parasympathetic nervous system is responsible for allowing sphincters to open and the release of bodily fluids. We need the parasympathetic system working well to allow for pooping, birthing, and orgasming with ease.

Keeping all of this in mind, you can see why choosing the place you feel the safest to birth is important. Just as you want your birth space to feel safe and soothing, you will also want your postpartum sanctuary space to feel safe so you can relax. You will have some unwinding to do from the birth experience, especially if things went unexpectedly, in either a heartbreaking or heartwarming way. A peaceful environment facilitates your nervous system's recalibration, and in turn encourages your milk to let down more quickly, ensuring an easier bond for the breastfeeding connection.

Another thing to consider is that interventions in the birth process affect our nervous system's functional capacity. When you are administered an anesthetic, it induces a freeze state in the body. Because the body is rendered immobile, even if only partially immobile, sympathetic responses are thwarted, meaning you can't move. If you cannot feel parts of your body and you could not move if you wanted to, the body perceives this as a danger. At a physiological level, this perception can correlate with a sense of helplessness and dissociation. On a practical level, this may add up to not being able to say what you want to say to your nurses, doctors, or midwives. You may feel confused or just simply "give up" on your birth plan or on advocating for your wishes.

The same is true for a surgical birth. While the anesthetic, in most cases, relieves or prevents pain, the body is still being cut, which is life-threatening. It is critical that women are able to complete the cycle produced by the anesthetic of imposed freeze followed by shaking as the medication leaves their system and their nervous system recalibrates— just like the rabbit's did. If you are reading this and it is resonating with you from your life experience or a birth experience, the section "Renegotiating a Birth That Needs Healing" in chapter 9 guides you through steps to begin to renegotiate your experience on your own.

ENJOYING EXPLORATORY SEX

What if I told you that sex could be just as good at preparing you for childbirth as childbirth-education classes are? Well, it's true.

Sex is one of the most fertile and unexplored territories of childbirth preparation. Opening up to exploring sex also sets couples up for a satisfying intimate life after the baby is born. An active, engaged sexual journey primes your body and mind for birth, motherhood, and a satisfying erotic life.

This is a sensitive topic, and I don't treat it lightly. Our culture's conversation regarding sex is so narrow that it is normal for us to experience a mixture of fascination and shame, discomfort and desire, attraction and aversion, when the topic arises. We encounter challenges in expressing ourselves, in having desire without guilt, with regard to our body image and our perception of what is sexy, attractive, and desirable. Many women I work with explain that they feel they understand the power of their sex but do not know how to access it. They feel there is a secret box that holds the keys to a transformative and even illuminated sex life, but they don't know how to get to them. This idea could be a whole book in itself, because sex is possibly the most potent and untapped tool for healing in our time, but there is a jumping-off point for how to deepen your sexuality while preparing for birth and after.

First, it's helpful to expand our definition of *sex* and understand a few things about the difference between male and female arousal.

Most people think of sex as penetration, known in the sex-education world as penis in vagina sex (PIV). When we define sex like this, it limits the way we connect and the possibility for new types of pleasure. When we only count sex as intercourse and climaxing, sex can become tally taking: I do you; then you do me. This is a limiting script. Women often feel guilty for taking too long. We fall into ruts, of actions or positions that we know we can orgasm in, and we don't necessarily explore different possibilities or ways we can experience pleasure.

Our cultural idea of sex is based on the male-arousal trajectory, which is a steady climb and then a sharp drop. This is what is typically portrayed when you see a man breathing and thrusting faster and faster, climaxing, and then falling asleep. Most porn is made for men, so even the women in porn are performing a male-arousal trajectory, building and building to a scream of a climax. But male and female arousal work differently.

Full arousal for men can take as little as thirty seconds to a minute. Female arousal works in rolling waves, ebbs and flows, and full arousal takes about thirty-five to forty-five minutes. This is the biology of how the erectile tissue works. For most women to get to a place where genital touch is a turn-on, it takes more time than it does for most men. While women have just as much engorgeable tissue as men (yes!), ours isn't nearly as visible, and is therefore more mysterious—to us and our partners. It's possible for women to have penetrative sex without being fully aroused, and enjoy it even. But penetration without full arousal becomes more difficult, and sometimes painful even, after having a baby. Although the changes in our sexuality can be disconcerting after birth, during the postpartum period there is a huge opportunity to expand our relationship to our own desires, erotic nature, and many new, undiscovered pleasure pathways.

Here are a few ways to expand erotic possibilities that can positively influence your birth experience.

Challenge Your Role as a Giver

Carve out time with your partner to practice receiving nongenital touch for fifteen or twenty minutes. Stick to just receiving, even if it is tempting to make it mutual. Experiment with different types and qualities of touch, such as tapping, light feather stroking, kneading, pinching, and using different body parts to touch with. Use a timer. Pause when the timer is finished and breathe together for one minute. Then, take the time to share one thing each of you learned or that was surprising. (If you are not partnered, you can do this with yourself—experiment with different kinds of touch, like kneading, tapping, patting, scratching on your own body.) If you are tempted to reciprocate or to only be the giver, resolve to change roles on another day. Allow yourself to exclusively receive, which is harder than it sounds for most of us.

Practice Using Your Voice

Allow yourself to make audible sounds. Get used to hearing unexpected sounds that arise from different sensations and from your unconscious. That way, when you are giving birth, your visceral sounds won't be as surprising.

Express what you like and what you don't like. If there's something you really don't like but have been tolerating, suggest an alternative. Develop your ability to say yes and no, and notice what doing so feels like in your body. If this is a challenging thing for you to do—and it is for most women—the word *maybe* may have to be *no* for a while. Get your partner involved by explaining that this is a process for you to get even more in touch with what you really want and love. Avoiding confusion and stopping yourself from the tendency to just go along with things will help you get clearer about what you want and find the power to express what you want—not just in the bedroom but also in your birth experience.

Sex without Sex

This one can be a bit of a hard sell, but it can also be a fascinating exercise that opens your mind and body to new sensations and experiences if you're willing to try it.

What would it be like to have an hour of sexual play with penetration and climax off the table? That might even sound confusing, because what are you doing sexually, for an hour, without the goal of trying to get the other person or yourself off? What if, instead, sex is about connecting and dropping everything, dropping all agendas? What if it is about following and deep listening? Can you be in the experience, rather than viewing the experience? Are you brave enough to experience the awkwardness of trying something new? If you do get close to a pleasure peak, can you go right to the edge of it, and then back off? Rather than going for the release, allow yourself to stay in the strong sensation, and dial it back. Slow everything way down. Be interested in micro movements. This is intimately connected to building your nervous-system capacity. When you are playing at the edges of your arousal, you are expanding the range of sensation that you can stay with, without going over the threshold into climax. This will help you expand your capacity for sensation

Expand Your Capacity for Sensation

Another way to expand your capacity for sensation is through sensory play. Assemble a basket with different objects like feathers, rocks, straws, oils, sandpaper, yarn, fur, and anything else with an interesting texture or smell. With eyes closed, pick up one of the objects and feel it in your hand. Imagine that you have never felt it before. After about thirty seconds, you will notice a shift. As you roll the object in your hand or slide it along your skin, instead of thinking about the object and making associations with it, you will actually sensorially perceive the object. It becomes infinitely more interesting. You can feel your hand and skin experiencing the object and you can feel the object itself. Continue for two minutes with the object; I like to set a timer, because two minutes can go by quickly or seem like forever. Be curious and find pleasure.

Identifying Your Core Erotic Theme

The idea of the core erotic theme comes from a book called the *Erotic Mind* by Jack Morin. He says, "Hidden within your Core Erotic Theme is a formula for transforming unfinished emotional business from childhood and adolescence into excitation and pleasure."

In this process of transforming unfinished emotional business, we can also be the protagonist of our erotic life and construct experiences that are deeply nourishing and satisfying. When we sit in a seat of empowerment with our sexuality, when we practice having and using a voice with our desires specifically related to our pelvis, we engage in magnificent birth and postpartum preparation practice.

Once you know at least one of your core erotic themes, you can take an active role in creating the kinds of sexual connection that you want to have. Some people worry that this might take the mystery out of connection. In fact, knowing a common thread between some of the highlights of your erotic life allows you to focus on experiences that have worked in the past, instead of what hasn't worked. This key also gives you another piece of self-knowledge to empower you to be proactive in the sex you want with tangible requests. Like most of these explorations, you can do them with a significant other or by yourself. If you have a good friend, you might want to suggest that you explore your core erotic themes together. Sometimes when you share the experiences, they can see commonalities that you can't. This can also be a great intimacy building practice to do with your partner. Each of you can write down your own experiences and then come together to share what you found. You don't have to share the details of the experiences, instead you can share the theme or themes you found and anything that surprised or interested you. Start this with an open mind and open heart. And if you are sharing with someone, suspend judgment and criticism; instead feel grateful that they are sharing something so intimate and vulnerable with you. This process is more linear than circular. It may take several times of circling back to the material and experiences that you retrieved to land on a theme. More information may come in your dreams now that you have begun the inquiry.

To discover your core erotic theme:

1. Brainstorm and write down three or four of your most erotic experiences. Don't judge yourself while doing so. This isn't a competition for the most outrageous or nastiest experiences you've ever had, although you may want to write those down and certainly can. This is about YOU. When you scan back through your sexual experiences, what stands out as exceptional? What grabs you?

2. After you have identified these experiences, go back and write about each one in detail. Describe, rather than analyze, the scene. Who was there? What was the environment like? What interesting details do you remember? Write in a way that someone who was not there could read it and get a sense of what it was like to be there. Tell the story of it.

3. Then, leave the writing overnight or for a day or even two. When you return, read through all of the descriptions. Use a pen to circle or underline key words that stand out as themes between the experiences, rather than within them. What is common to the experiences that you chose? (This step can be hard to do alone. If you have a girlfriend that is willing to go through the process with you, you could read them to each other. Someone else is often able to see themes that we may not see.)

4. After you find clues about a theme, reflect on your current sexual self. Is your erotic theme currently being incorporated into and attended to in your intimate life?

5. Homework: Design a self-pleasure practice that includes an element of your core erotic theme.
6. Extra credit: Invite your partner into an experience that includes a part of your theme.

Building the Buffet

Start a list of your sexual desires. You may begin with what you learned from your core erotic theme to build a treasure trove of your fantasies and ideas about your erotic life. This can be anything from taking a bath with your partner to an evening under the stars to wanting to experiment with a specific sexual position. In my practice, I have noticed that this is a difficult practice for most people to even begin. In our culture, the dialogue about sex is usually limited to frequency (how often?) or technique, sex acts or positions.

If you want to include frequency or acts that you are curious about on your list, that's great. Also include ways that you would like to feel during sex and curiosities you might have about your own body, your partner's body, and the fantasies each of you have. I suggest that you each write down your own list and then compare notes, adding them together to create a joint buffet. Know that you don't have to act these out, although you may want to. Build intimacy by sharing and exploring desires that may seem weird or taboo. Everyone's idea of taboo is different. I have worked with couples who were too embarrassed and afraid to share their desires for years, only to find out when they did that they were shared. What sweet relief! However, even if they are not shared, there is intimacy in the sharing without judgment. (Note that if you or your partner watch a lot of porn, it will influence your or their fantasies. If only one partner is watching porn, the other is often less receptive to the fantasies the other expresses, especially if the partner can tell the fantasies are coming from porn, which seem manufactured rather than authentic desires.)

Giving birth and the journey of motherhood require losing control on a physical and emotional level. How do you prepare to lose control? You practice losing it just a little bit at a time. Receiving, relaxing about the outcome, expanding your capacity to feel, and being inside the experience will all help you surf the waves of arousal, orgasm, and surging contractions. If you are in a sexual routine, this is a great time to explore sex in a way that will prepare you for birth and expand the possibilities of intimacy and growth. A richer and more diverse sexual connection that explores new pleasure pathways will be an exceptional foundation for the rebirth of your sexual connection postpartum.

SUMMARY

- In preparing your body for birth, stay or get active, but do not overdo it. Listen to your body and your health-care professionals about exercise.
- Practice gentle exercises and stretching that will help you give birth, therefore aiding your postpartum recovery as well.
- Remember that stability is compromised by loose ligaments so watch overstretching and overloading your joints.
- You can practice letting your pelvic floor open up and you can manually stretch your perineal muscles.
- Cross-train your nervous system by alternating between phases of activation and relaxation, doing and being.
- Expanding your sexuality can be an amazing way to prepare for giving birth.

Practices
- Practice the breath for length two minutes a day.
- Download the audio to learn how to do a proper Kegel for birth preparation and recovery (at www.magamama.com/pelvic-mapping). Practice at least once.

- If you are a yogini, gymnast, horseback rider, or Pilates or barre-method enthusiast, emphasize the pushing action of pelvic-floor movement. Consider scheduling a pelvic-health session with a physical therapist or sexological bodyworker for help releasing your pelvic floor before giving birth.
- If you have a history of sexual abuse or hospital trauma, invest in a doula and somatic therapy, such as trauma resolution through Somatic Experiencing, to facilitate your birth process and consequently your postpartum experience.
- Take at least one step outside of your sexual routine by practicing one of the exercises listed above.

Reflections

- Notice where you are in the spectrum of activity—too much or too little—and seek to move toward balance.
- Make a list of curiosities or desires about your own body, your partner's body, and ways you would like to explore.
- Write down three or four of your most erotic experiences and identify your core erotic themes. Then go back and look at what they have in common. Now create a scenario that includes some of those elements.

Part Two

SAVORING THE
FOURTH TRIMESTER

.... 🌿 ....

The moment a child is born, the mother is also born.
She never existed before.
The woman existed, but the mother never.
A mother is something absolutely new.

—OSHO

Congratulations! You did it. You crossed the threshold. You birthed a baby, and you birthed yourself into a new phase of life. There is no more pronounced shift in body, mind, and spirit than becoming a mother. The transition to motherhood, which is ongoing and individual, requires respect. Cultures all over the world have honored the time following birth by allowing new mothers to rest, feeding them nutritious food, and offering healing hands.

This sacred window, as it is called in India, is a time you want to savor. Though it is a relatively short time, it can offer huge rewards. Rest and be nourished and you will not only experience a deep abiding bliss now, but you will take that with you and set yourself up for true health throughout the rest of your motherhood journey and your life as well. Savoring the sacred window can seem difficult and even overwhelming at times, anathema to the way we have operated before. For one, it can seem impossible to expect to rest when we have a newborn, especially when, in the hours and days directly after giving birth, our emotions can be hard to get a handle on (and by handle, I don't mean controlling them so much as understanding them).

That is why we start part two discussing commonly covered issues like "baby blues," postpartum depression, and hormones. Before you get overwhelmed by the information out there, it's good to know what is normal and can simply be "ridden out" by accepting these fluctuations as par for the course.

And though resting and nourishing ourselves with a newborn can seem like a herculean task, this part will go through specific tools and suggestions that will help you attend to the five universal post-partum needs—rest, nourishing food, loving touch, spiritual companionship, and contact with nature—to help you come through this time fortified and whole.

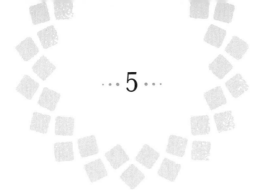

balancing your emotions

Giving birth and becoming a mother may be one of the biggest transitions you ever experience. While your baby is now outside your body, there is still an intricate connection between the two of you. Your energy and emotional systems are not yet separate and won't be for a while. To set the stage for a satisfying and even blissful recovery, make choices that reflect your delicate, new relationship. Your baby's nervous system is developing now, and yours is recalibrating. Having your home as calm and peaceful as possible will provide the ideal sanctuary at this time. On every level, you are adapting to an enormous cascade of changes—energetically, hormonally, structurally, and organically—in a short period of time. Swells of emotion, while they can be unpredictable and disconcerting, are absolutely normal at this time. This chapter will give you the nuts and bolts of what you need to understand about your hormones and emotions during this transition.

PROTECTING THE MOTHERBABY

There is a word in Swahili, *mamatoto*, which means "motherbaby." This word reflects the understanding that, in the early postpartum months, mother and baby are interconnected and interdependent physically, energetically, and spirituality.

Similarly, Argentinian psychologist Laura Gutman uses the terms *mommybaby* and *babymommy* to emphasize that, while now physically separate, a baby and its mother are still so connected in the months after birth that using separate words to define them doesn't work. Mother and baby are still intricately linked and do not exist without each other. They are defined by one another. A baby's health depends on its mother; a mother's health depends on her baby. The baby is a reflection of its mother's psyche and is defined only in relationship to its environment that, early on, is mother. This interdependent union is different from any other bond. As such, it has specific and basic instructions dictated as much by physiology as by intuition or ancestral wisdom.

Even our term *fourth trimester* suggests a time where the baby is as dependent on the mother as it was during the first three trimesters. Of course, after birth, the baby is separate from us physically. However, as Laura Gutman describes in *Maternity, Coming Face to Face with Your Own Shadow*:

> This newly born body is not just substance. A subtle, spiritual body exists as well. While physical separation does take place, a bond belonging to another plane persists. Even while separated, the newborn and his mother remain in a state of emotional fusion. This infant emerged from his mother's physical and spiritual viscera and is still a part of the emotional surroundings in which he was submerged. While development of the intellect has not yet begun, the infant preserves subtle intuitive and telepathic skills that utterly bind him to his mother's soul.

Some care is now being taken to ease the abrupt transition for the baby from inner world to outer world. More hospitals allow babies to stay in the room after birth and encourage skin-to-skin contact. Lotus birth, where the umbilical cord is not cut and the placenta is left intact after the birth, has become more popular as a way to honor the connection and soften disruption of that connection. Nevertheless, the physical separation occurs, while emotional and spiritual fusion remain.

Because this interconnectedness seems so miraculous and a bit foreign to us, videos circulate on social media about women whose babies were not breathing but then "came to life" when kept in contact with their mothers. Of course a new baby would be recharged and revived by its mother, the source of its physical, emotional, and spiritual life. I have witnessed the power of this motherbaby connection in reverse.

Community Stories:
Alison

It's not just babies who need their mothers or can be revived by them. Alison, a mother for whom I served as a doula, had a C-section and her baby was taken to the observation nursery immediately afterward. I went with Alison from the operating room back to her recovery room. Minutes and then hours went by as she waited for her baby. She continued moaning as if contracting and began to wail, describing the pain as worse than her labor pain. The nurses kept coming in to increase the dosage of her pain medication. Nothing was providing relief. Sensing that her body was yearning for her baby and distraught at how long her perfectly healthy baby was being "observed," I kept calling the nursery asking for him to be brought back up to her room. I held her hand as she screamed and cried in anguish, pleading for more pain meds, but there was nothing more they could give her. Sure enough, the moment her baby was brought to her, her pain subsided. She immediately stopped crying and the contractions waned.

A mother's body needs her new baby. Physically, energetically, and spiritually, there is a rupture when a new baby is taken far away from its mother and vice versa, so we must do our best to heed the wisdom of the motherbaby, to create conditions for the motherbaby to thrive.

An unwanted separation of mother and baby after delivery creates an enormous amount of stress on both the mother and the baby. This stress can create difficulty for bonding and breastfeeding. When mother and baby are together after a physiological birth, these initial hours have been called the golden hours, because of the surge of love hormones that floods the atmosphere, blessing everyone in it. The nervous systems of mother and the baby are signaling each other, conveying levels of safety or levels of stress.

Interventions like medication or mechanical or surgical delivery interrupt the motherbaby field. A difficult or traumatic delivery is also a rupture to the motherbaby system. Chapter 9 gives more specific instructions on how to work with births that need healing.

One way to support the thriving of the motherbaby unit is to make sure that the energy of the birth process is complete. It will help the mother to feel more grounded, oriented, and present, so she can respond and attune to her baby's evolving needs.

Completing the Birth Energy

Just as we have physical bodies made of bones, muscles, and joints, we also have energetic bodies. The energetic body cannot be touched directly, but it can be felt. This powerful circuitry is what both yoga and traditional Chinese medicine work to affect. They unblock stuck energy passing through these channels and strengthen our ability to carry energy through our system, so our immune, endocrine, and nervous systems are hearty and resilient.

The raw energy of birth is magnificent. In order to access and channel the power and force necessary to give birth, a woman's energy fields expand. Paralleling the downward physical movement required to push a baby out, birth energy moves from top to bottom during birth. Women are pulling cosmic energy down through their bodies, into the earthly, material realm.

The birth process itself is a powerful downward process, and this forceful downward movement requires that both the physical body and the energetic body open to a greater degree than ever before. The lower energy centers are opened to near maximum. Just as many women may not have considered the physical impact that this process may set in motion, most of us haven't considered what will happen from an energetic standpoint either.

While it can seem vague and intangible, especially in a culture that does not include the language of energy and spirit in most health conversations, the expansion of the energy field and its changed shape in the birth process is real. After giving birth, women need to first complete the birth energy, helping it flow all the way through their systems. Then they need to assist their energy field in returning to a comfortable size. The visualizations, "Completing the Birth Cycle" and "Shrinking the Birth Field," guide you in creating these shifts to preserve motherbaby harmony.

We may be unaccustomed to acknowledging the power of our energy field, but working with it has tangible effects. As a bodyworker, I combine energy work with physical touch to help women complete the birth-energy cycle. The motherbaby physiology is designed for unmedicated vaginal birth. Therefore when births take other directions, there are often unfinished physiological processes that parallel the unfinished energetic processes. I have worked on many women who have delivered babies via cesarean section and even up to fifteen years post-birth when I touch their scar, they have experienced the taste of anesthetic, the anger at a flippant or unkind doctor, and the excruciating sensation of not being numb enough on one side of the incision when going back into the birth experience. It's also not uncommon for women who delivered via C-section to experience uterine contractions during this process. The body has cellular memory of birth as a downward process with uterine contractions, cervical expansion, and stretching of the vaginal tissues. When birth happens another way, the body's physiological memory is thwarted.

Babies who are born via cesarean section or with mechanical help, such as with forceps or vacuum extraction, also often have unfinished movements. They weren't able to do the pushing movement with their feet, the first movement of spinal extension under the pubic bone, or receive the cranial massage from the pressure of the vaginal walls. These reflexes and impulses are a very important beginning part of human development. There are many modalities that specialize in helping babies recover these steps, including BodyMind Centering, Biodynamic Craniosacral work, the Anat Baniel method, Feldenkrais, and Somatic Experiencing. Giving babies support in completing their birth experience can affect everything from colic and sleep patterns in the short term to motor skills and emotional development in the long term.

Whatever kind of birth you had, whether heartening or heartbreaking, or somewhere in between, engage this simple process of completing the birth cycle to give all parts of you the chance to move forward together into the sacred window.

COMPLETING THE BIRTH CYCLE

Begin with an intention and a prayer. Lodge this prayer in your mind, heart, and womb space. Ask that light or spirit or God remove all that does not belong to you. Ask grace to help release the birth energy and whatever is in its way, moving it down and out. Acknowledge its power and all the ways it helped you. Visualize a stream of bright light passing from your crown down through all of energy centers and out through your vagina, clearing whatever is in the way of this light traveling freely through. Allow whatever is old, unnecessary, or not yours to go with the light out and down into the earth. You can begin this process two to three days after the birth, and continue daily for the first two weeks. But you can also do this anytime. If you are reading this book years after giving birth, I suggest that you call to mind a memory from when you gave birth. Call that memory forth in your body, and when that moment is clear in your mind's eye, call in the divine energy or life force and allow it to move through you.

During birth, your energy field expanded as much as it probably ever will in your life. That expanded field is helpful in allowing you to open to greater wisdom and strength than normally available. For day-to-day life and new mothering, it is important to restore your energy field to a manageable size.

SHRINKING THE BIRTH FIELD

- Close your eyes and imagine the space that you are occupying and your energy field. There is no right or wrong here. Feel into it intuitively. Feel your physical body and then your energy body all around you.
- Imagine this light-space shrinking and coming closer, back toward your skin, until you can feel yourself in an egg-shaped container of light that is protective and nurturing.
- Imagine this dense and loving golden light is nourishing you with the love and connection that you need.
- And then move one more layer in, toward your skin, and imagine being lightly draped in a gossamer net. Feel the contours of your skin and relax into your own body. Your intention to return to the material realm through your physical body will help ground you.

What is required energetically at birth—expansiveness, transcendence, and openness—is quite different from what is required of women postpartum—presence, groundedness, steadfastness. If we can gently assist our energy field in returning to a comfortable size and guide the birth energy out and through, we will experience more focused awareness and less overall confusion and disorientation.

In addition to the size of the birth field changing, the concentration and distribution of energy also changes during birth. The upper centers, which connect us to universal energy, become open and receptive. The lower centers also become supercharged, connecting us to the earth, our ancestry, and to our basic sense of safety and belonging. The energy center at our solar plexus, the place of individual expression, shrinks as we give life to another being. At the moment of giving birth, our energy system forms an hourglass configuration; we are highly receptive to transcendental connection and available for an experience of universal consciousness—we have a wide-open crown. At the moment we are bringing life into the world, we are offered the possibility of entering into contact with the source of life itself. Likewise, at the base we are wide open. We are offered the opportunity to connect to the earth, the ground of being, our physical home.

The process of consolidating our energy postpartum requires that we seal the energy at the pelvis and the crown of the head. When the energy centers are dialed open, they are more vulnerable and exposed. As part of the reintegration process after birth, the lower two centers corresponding to the pelvic floor, cervix, and womb need support to come back into balance as well. This is true no matter how the birth went. Often if women have had a revelatory birth experience, there may be an inner hesitancy to seal their system back up, lest they lose contact with the bliss and transcendence that they encountered during the birth. On the other hand, if a woman had a difficult birth experience, the two lower chakras may seem vague and distant.

In yoga, major energy centers are called *chakras*, from the Sanskrit word that means "circle" or "wheel." They are located along the spine and correspond to nerve plexes in the physical body. They are associated with emotional and spiritual qualities. In most systems there are seven of them. The first chakra is the root, located for women either at the perineum or the cervix, related to the whole pelvic floor. It is associated with stability, security, and connection to our tribe. The second chakra in women is located in the womb and the sacrum. It is the center of our creativity and sexuality. The first and second chakras are the energy centers that are most affected by birth, as birth occurred in their territory.

Whatever unresolved experiences, physical or energetic, that have lingered in that territory can be shaken loose and reactivated during birth. The seventh chakra, or crown chakra, relates to our connection to our higher selves and to the Divine.

The necessity for protecting and sealing the lower energy centers is consistent with the way that many cultures use heat and contact after birth to cocoon the mother (see more in the "Mother Warming" section in chapter 6). In East Africa, many women sit over scalding hot steam right after giving birth. From a Western medical perspective, that would be seen as creating more blood flow and potentially leading to swelling. However, this East African practice uses heat to help seal the energy openings. The belly wrapping used in countries all over the world, from Java to Brazil, has both physical and energetic purposes. The *rebozo*, a fabric wrap from Mexico, is used not just to help a woman's organs be firm and protected, but also to give a woman a sense of her personal boundaries. Many cultures insist that new mothers stay indoors and limit visitors, so that they have time to harmonize their physical and energetic bodies.

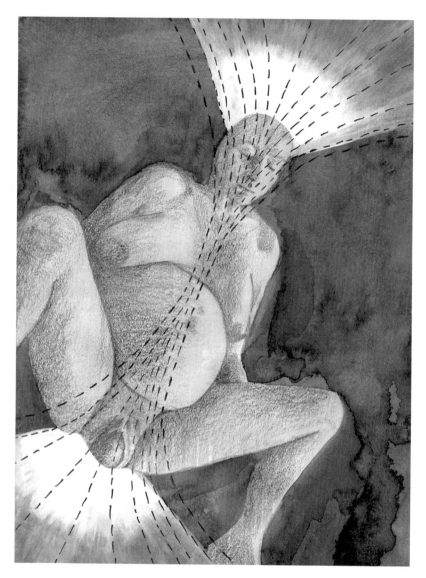

Fig. 9: Birth hourglass

If the birth experience organizes our energy body like an hourglass (fig. 9), the postpartum reorganization looks like a seedpod (fig. 10). We begin to close up the top and the bottom, the crown and the root, so we can reconnect with our own sense of personal identity in our middle centers. We are learning how to feel ourselves as an individual

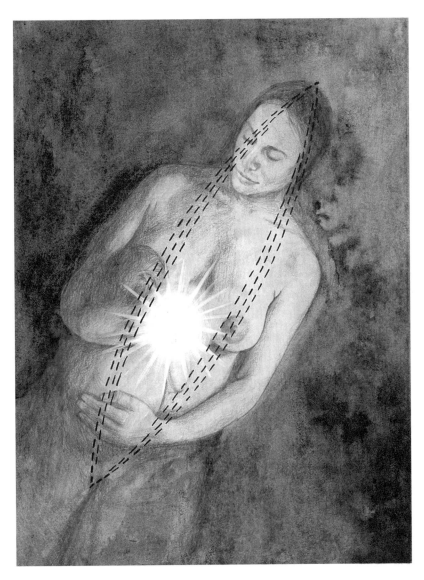

Fig. 10: Birth seedpod

while at the same time being intimately connected to another individual. This transition will happen on its own as it follows the natural fluctuation of how all of life works, a constant pulse between expansion and contraction; however, if we are aware of this process as it is happening, we can encourage and savor each stage.

Honoring Your Womb Space

There are some symbolic gestures that we can take as remembrances of the sacred power of our womb that just birthed life. Especially at this time of purification, restoration, and renewal after childbirth, it is strengthening to have reminders of the power of all of life that is born through the womb space. I suggest that each new mom choose a bowl to eat from that is hers only. The bowl itself is a symbol of the womb. Committing to being sustained from this bowl and not sharing what is in it allows a new mother to maintain a sense of dignity and boundaries. This is not a denial of the motherbaby, but a nod to the need for us to be sustained and nurtured, so we can stay tuned in. As mothers, we share and give so much that it is important to maintain our individuality in small yet significant ways. Another suggestion is to have a bowl with water and a flower in it on your bedside table, mantel, or altar space.

WHAT EXACTLY IS HAPPENING WITH MY HORMONES?

Of course, the changes we experience during pregnancy and birth encompass more than physical and energetic changes: they also include hormonal changes. During pregnancy, you not only grew a baby inside you, but you also grew an organ—the placenta. After you deliver the placenta, your hormones start to shift dramatically. In the first day or two after delivery, you will probably experience an exhilarating high. No matter how your baby was born, what satisfaction and accomplishment it is to finally meet your baby! It is normally after the first forty-eight hours, as the endorphins start to wear off, that women begin to experience fluctuations in moods and emotions. This is what is labeled the "baby blues." Because there is so much information and fear out there about postpartum depression, many women panic, thinking that this weepy time will last forever. For most women, these cascading emotions normalize at around two weeks postpartum.

From the time the placenta was birthed to when breast milk comes in, a woman's estrogen and progesterone levels plummet to the levels of a menopausal woman. Progesterone, the calm and chill hormone that you became accustomed to in pregnancy, goes offline, so the hormones needed for breastfeeding can come online more quickly. The process of hormonal calibration continues for months, as the body works to get the uterus back to normal size and to produce an increasing amount of breast milk for a growing baby. The body is flushing itself of excess fluids that store now-unnecessary hormones. One of the reasons that new mothers are encouraged to stay warm and sweat a lot (see "Mother Warming" in chapter 6) is so this process of flushing can be thorough and complete. Tears can also be a part of this process of elimination.

Rather than understanding the role of each specific hormone, it is important to understand how they work in coordination with each other. For this purpose, I love the way that Dr. Claudia Welch, in her book *Balance Your Hormones, Balance Your Life*, divides hormones into two categories: *yin* sex hormones and *yang* stress hormones. Our body only has so much energy and raw material with which to create hormones. Because our survival is the fundamental need, our body will always prioritize the making of stress hormones that are critical to our survival. Many things register as a greater threat to our nervous system than they actually are. Perceived threat results in a cascade of stress hormones being released. If we are under stress, our body will direct resources to our survival responses, which are related to stress, rather than to our pleasure and sex circuitry, which is related to our ability to relax, bond, and breastfeed.

Fortunately the converse is also true: if sex hormones are being produced, the body is less likely to produce stress hormones. So if a woman feels safe, secure, and protected, her body will produce the sex hormones that reinforce this feeling of relaxation, which, in turn, helps with milk production and the healing process.

The Hormones You Need to Know About

Sex Hormones

The sex hormones are the feel-good hormones. Women's dominant sex hormones are estrogen and progesterone. Both are produced in the ovaries until, early in the second trimester of pregnancy, the placenta takes over the hormone production and they are produced by the placenta.

Estrogen is the juiciest female hormone, giving women our trademark sex characteristics, like voluptuous breasts, wide hips, and full lips. During pregnancy, estrogen maintains the strong uterine lining, increases the blood circulation, and acts as the master regulator of the other key hormones. After giving birth, estrogen levels drop and stay low for as long as a woman is breastfeeding. Estrogen is found in every tissue of the body and is responsible for lubrication.

Progesterone is estrogen's counterpart. A woman's progesterone levels increase to up to two hundred times their normal levels during pregnancy. So it is a steep drop when progesterone leaves the body after the delivery of the placenta, allowing milk production to begin. After the baby is born and the placenta is delivered, the ovaries need to take over the job of producing progesterone again. Progesterone is what gives some pregnant women a happy, dreamy, even-keeled emotional state; the sharp decrease in progesterone can leave a new mom feeling like she has less resilience to all the changes postpartum. Progesterone only returns to a normal level when a woman begins ovulating.

Oxytocin has been called the "love hormone" and the "cuddle hormone." It promotes attachment and bonding. Oxytocin is released after a thirty-second hug, and also while watching cute puppy or baby videos. Oxytocin is responsible for the fetal ejection reflex, uterine contractions during birth, and the special bonding that occurs between all of the people who are present at the birth. Touch is one of the best ways to encourage oxytocin and why new moms need as much loving touch as they are offering to their new babies.

Relaxin is produced at ten times its normal rate during pregnancy, so ligaments and joints soften, making space in the pelvis for the baby to come out. Because relaxin affects all the joints, some women may experience pain in other joints in the body, as they become looser and less stable. As long as women are breastfeeding, relaxin will continue to be produced in the body, so joints and ligaments may not return to their most strong and stable place until after breastfeeding has been stopped.

Stress Hormones

Stress hormones aren't all bad. They help to accelerate some fetal development as well as give women the added energy needed to push a baby out! But most often, we are producing way more stress hormones than we need, and that blocks us from accessing the positive, nurturing sex hormones that we need to experience a pleasant, even blissful, postpartum period.

Adrenaline and *cortisol* work together. Adrenaline is responsible for a short-term burst of fight-or-flight energy that then quickly decreases. Cortisol is always released with adrenaline but is longer acting and, therefore, has longer-lasting effects.

During pregnancy, cortisol increases, especially during the last trimester. This is thought to help speed fetal lung and brain development just before birth. After childbirth, while it is mostly the sex hormones that are responsible for milk production and letdown, some cortisol is also needed. Too much cortisol, though, will compete with the sex hormones, contribute to anxiety and stress, and block access to the oxytocin circuitry that can make the milk letdown of breastfeeding feel relaxing and pleasurable.

The practices given in the "Cross-Training Your Nervous System" section of chapter 4 have given you a felt sense of what these hormonal upswings and downswings feel like in your nervous system. Under stress, when you imagined losing your car keys, cortisol started coursing through your veins, your heart pumped faster, you may have started to sweat. Recalling your favorite vacation spot allowed you to exhale and slow down. These practices also give you a way to reconnect to the present moment through your senses, which is one key to generating more sex hormones.

Asking for Blood Work

Just as it is a proactive step in your health care to schedule a postpartum visit with a physical therapist, it is also wise to ask your ob-gyn at your six-week checkup for a full blood panel to check your hormone levels and immune function. Because antidepressants and birth control pills are often blanket prescriptions in women's health, underlying hormonal or immune system imbalances may be missed and left untreated. This situation can be avoided by simply asking for blood work at your doctor visit.

It is especially important to check your hormone levels before considering taking antidepressants, so you are treating the right problem. I have recently seen an increasing number of women in my practice who have developed autoimmune disorders in the postpartum period. Many women experience a significant difference in thyroid function after having a baby. A staggering one in twelve postpartum women is diagnosed with Hashimoto's disease, an autoimmune disorder of the thyroid. Under-functioning thyroid and adrenal glands can present much like depression. The blood work can also show you how your body is processing cortisol.

While a stress response to an event as big as birth is normal, this healthy amount of stress can be mitigated when a postpartum mother is bathed in sex hormones. The "baby blues" can be less blue if a woman is surrounded by people who love her and she is receiving love through delicious food and caring touch.

To understand more about the role of hormones and how to work with them holistically, I highly recommend the book *WomanCode* by Alisa Vitti. This book was so instrumental in my own healing process that I asked Alisa to write the foreword for this book. Her website, FLOLiving.com, is an accessible resource that provides hormonal support postpartum and beyond so that you can easily understand the steps it takes to balance your hormones with nutrition and lifestyle changes. Implementing the five-step protocol, which has helped many women heal from gynecological challenges including painful periods to polycystic ovarian syndrome to fertility challenges, is an accessible step to balancing your hormones postpartum.

If you need more help and support, the next step is to request bloodwork from your ob-gyn, a naturopath or a functional medicine doctor. Knowing what is happening with your physiology, with respect to immunity and thyroid function, is important before landing on diagnoses of depression.

SUMMARY

- While a mother and baby physically separate at birth, their energy and emotional systems are still intricately interconnected.
- After you deliver the placenta, your hormone levels drop dramatically and begin a months' long process of recalibration from growing and birthing a baby to now nursing a baby and helping your body recover.
- Between forty-eight hours and two weeks postpartum it is normal to be weepy and emotional, also known as the "baby blues."

- Sometimes hormone imbalances, autoimmune disorders, isolation, and lack of support can look like depression.

Reflections

- Are there parts of you that feel left behind in the birth experience? Do you feel that your baby was able to complete his or her birth process?
- What is the experience like for you to be physically separate yet very emotionally and energetically connected to your baby now?
- In what ways can you honor and stay connected to your womb space?

Practices

- Do the exercise "Completing the Birth Cycle." This and the following exercise are inspired by the work of Tami Lynn Kent, a women's health physical therapist who developed a practice of physical-energetic tools to better access the medicine of the pelvic bowl called holistic pelvic care. She is the author of *Wild Feminine* and other books and teaches this practice (see www.wildfeminine .com for more information).
- Do the exercise "Shrinking the Birth Field."
- Before taking the pill or antidepressants, ask your ob-gyn or a naturopath for a blood-work panel to check your hormones and your immune-system function.

restoring your vitality

For three years after I had my daughter, I kept trying to turn myself into an ideal of what health looked like. I wanted to feel better, so I would exercise. Without fail, I would feel more exhausted instead of energized, which was the opposite of how things had always worked for me. Before every menstrual cycle, I would have an allergy attack that led to a cold that led to a sinus infection. I was so frustrated with this cycle of illness that I sought help from an acupuncturist who practiced traditional Chinese medicine. After a few sessions, he told me that I absolutely had to prioritize two things— eating and resting. That was it.

When I was not caring for my daughter or working, I needed to rest. During any free moments at all, I needed to lie down. He asked me to minimize time outside my house and trips around the city, staying close to home to cook for myself, eat regularly, and sleep. Apart from my work teaching yoga classes and giving private yoga sessions, the only thing I could do was gentle breathing exercises. After years of spending my days in almost constant motion, practicing yoga, teaching yoga, and using yoga and dance to manage my energy and health, now I was being advised to do absolutely nothing. His advice was counterintuitive to what I knew created a healthy lifestyle. If I hadn't been so exhausted from repeatedly experiencing these cycles of illness, and if I hadn't trusted this acupuncturist so much, I probably wouldn't have heeded his advice.

In the end, I was so glad I did. The postpartum time requires a radical shift in energy for most of us, one that brings a whole new rhythm to our lives. As we've touched on before, in our society we have idealized inexhaustible energy, the kind that can squeeze work, exercise, and meditation, as well as family and social relationships, all into a typical day. Yet most of us, even those who don't have children, seem to be scrambling to find balance.

Ayurveda and classical Chinese medicine offer time-honored wisdom for finding that balance and, in particular, wisdom for the postpartum period that helps women truly restore their vitality, rebuild their systems, and emerge even stronger after having children. To our grandmothers and great-grandmothers, it was normal and acceptable to slow down after having a baby. That wisdom can be rediscovered, and we can look to the Eastern traditions for that guidance and for discovering how to honor this special time in our lives.

Both the Ayurvedic and Chinese medicine perspectives on postpartum health could be volumes on their own. I have tried to offer the most elemental concepts, everything from Chinese medicine's view of the elements, fluids, chi flow, and diet as well as Ayurvedic doshas, body types, and asanas. The systems share the foundational principles of postpartum care such as a harmonious environment, good company, nutrient rich whole foods, and mother warming or roasting. If the specificities of each system get overwhelming, return to the basic principles. Implementing them will enhance the quality of your postpartum window as well as your life beyond.

NOURISHING YIN

Classical Chinese medicine recognizes that life transitions are vulnerable times and should be supported with special attention and care. The time after a woman gives birth is seen as the biggest transition that a woman can go through in her entire life—bigger than a woman's own birth, menarche, or menopause.

Chinese medicine considers a woman to be in an imbalanced state postpartum, and the quality of her recovery influences her health for the rest of her life. During the postpartum time, you can restore your health, both past issues as well as post-birth problems, by following the principles of Chinese medicine with respect to lifestyle and diet. However, if one breaks the rules of sitting out the month/moon, illnesses can become deeply entrenched in the body and even intensify years later.

Sun Simiao, the great Tang dynasty scholar and physician, wrote extensively on gynecology. He viewed women's health as central to a healthy society, which was radical in 700 A.D. Sabine Welms's translation of Sun Simiao's work *Essential Prescriptions* states, "He included the female body in the larger perspective of life beyond just the individual body, as well as the survival of the family for generations to come, and ultimately the altruistic ideal of benefiting society and the macrocosm at large." Sun Simiao "eloquently argued for the need for 'separate prescriptions' and special care for women's bodies and minds" and concluded that women are "ten times more difficult to treat" than men. This is due to the intricacy of our monthly cycles, our birthing cycles, and the entire life cycle of shifts in our endocrine and reproductive systems.

Understanding the uniqueness of a woman's biological and energetic makeup makes the postpartum time in a woman's life highly respected and revered. After a woman makes such an enormous donation of energy in birthing a child, she is protected, served, and nurtured in body, mind, and spirit. Her family, community, and entire cultural system are oriented toward helping her replenish what has been lost, so she may return to robust health and fulfill her role in society as a mother. Of course, each woman will experience this time differently, but Chinese medicine offers some very useful principles to help us understand what our systems undergo during and after birth.

The Fluids of Chinese Medicine

Nourishing your yin, blood, and chi are important aspects of restoring your vitality, but what are they exactly? Let's start with *yin*.

Yin

Yin and yang are opposite, complementary forces that are defined by their relationship and proportion to one another. If yin refers to the shadow side of a mountain, then yang represents the sunny side. As the earth turns and shifts its position to the sun, how much we see of either side of the mountain changes. So there is always a dynamic balance of these two forces.

Yin qualities are watery, dark, cold, slow, and moist. Yang qualities are fiery, bright, hot, fast, and dry. Yin is nighttime; yang is daytime. Yin is considered female and connected to the archetypal feminine. Yang is considered male and connected to the archetypal masculine. Blood and essence (*jing*) is yin, and life force (chi) is yang. The front of the body, the inner arms and legs, and the perineum are yin; the back of the body, the outer arms and legs, and the top of the head are yang. Mothers are yin; children are yang.

Pregnancy is primarily a yin state of being, while birth is a dynamic balance of yin and yang. When uninterrupted, much of labor happens at night, when the atmosphere is quiet, dark, and yin in nature. Childbirth involves lots of bodily fluids, also yin. But yang is also necessary in labor, as expressed through the force and intensity of the muscular movement of the uterus as it pushes the baby and the placenta out. Because birth creates a yin deficiency in the loss of blood and fluid, there is an imbalance after birth. Having a baby exaggerates the tendencies that are already present in a woman's system; if a woman is already yin deficient, then she will have the tendency to become even more yin deficient after having a baby. Because most of our lifestyles are yang dominant, many women are yin deficient.

YIN	YANG
shadow side of the mountain	sunny side of the mountain
watery	fiery
dark	bright
cold	hot
slow	fast
moist	dry
nighttime	daytime
blood and jing (essence)	chi (see below)
perineum	top of the head
feminine	masculine
mothers	children
sex hormones	stress hormones

Chi

What is chi? The word *chi* is usually translated as "vital energy." In English, the word *energy* is pretty vague. It can refer to everything from vibes, as in "that person has toxic energy," to power sources, such as "solar energy," to our own level of vigor, "I'm feeling drained of energy today." Chi, however, describes the animating, primordial force of the universe present in all things.

One of the main objectives of acupuncture is to harmonize the flow of chi through our bodies' meridians, which are the distribution network of chi, blood, and other fluids, and to heal and optimize organ health. Blockages in the meridians cause pain and prevent the free flow of chi and blood. Free-flowing chi in the meridians gives one a warm, glowing feeling and is a sign of radiant health.

Blood

In Chinese medicine, *blood* is both the actual fluid that we know as blood and the underlying activating energy that stimulates blood to move and circulate throughout the body. Blood and chi are interconnected. Chi moves the blood, and blood cannot be formed without chi. It is said that "blood is the mother of chi. Chi is the commander of blood." Because physical, mental, and spiritual health are interconnected in this worldview, blood is considered to be the substance of the body that grounds the spirit. When blood is ample, the spirit is quiet—another compelling reason to build blood. Women need to take care of the state of their blood (which is yin in nature, in contrast to the yang nature of chi) in order to be healthy.

During childbirth, all women will experience a loss of chi and blood. The channels of the mother are open, and disease factors (such as cold, wind, damp, heat, and dryness) can penetrate deeply into the body and cause illness. In the West, these concepts are just beginning to come into our cultural consciousness, but Eastern tradition offers simple and trusted ways for a new mother to nourish yin, build her blood, and revitalize chi so she may return to total health. Food is medicine, so we begin with food nourishment.

Food as Medicine

To nourish blood, yin, and essence, we need rest, mineral- and collagen-rich foods, and emotional and spiritual comfort—a close parallel to the five universal postpartum needs! Traditionally, herbal formulas and food choices for postpartum mothers are designed to be deeply nourishing on many levels, replenishing blood, chi, yin, yang, and body fluids.

To counteract the cold of blood deficiency, a new mother will benefit from eating warming foods and foods that build blood. These include:
- Beef
- Chicken
- Eggs
- Black sesame seeds
- Dates

- Cooked greens
- Carrots
- Soups

Note: A more complete grocery list to help you stock your pantry and orient your friends to what kind of food you would like can be found in appendix 5.

The focus of the first two weeks is completing the cleansing of the uterus, minimizing risk of infection, and aiding milk production. Special but simple soups can be made during these first two weeks to help complete bleeding, which is the elimination process that cleanses the uterus as it returns to its normal size. A famous Chinese herbal formula designed for postpartum women is called Engender and Transform Decoction (Sheng Hua Tang). This formula is designed to help expel old blood from the uterus while helping form new, healthy blood. It helps to reduce infection and promote breast-milk production. No single formula is the right one for everyone, so it is wise to consult a Chinese medicine practitioner to customize your treatment.

In the subsequent weeks, soups and stews change in their objective from detoxification to fortification; now they are made to strengthen chi and blood. The tonic soups can be continued to help ensure high-quality breast milk, which is formed from the mother's blood and chi.

In traditional Chinese medicine, emotional blockages (such as resentment and anger) can easily become physical ones, like mastitis, so emotional stability and a gentle environment are also important to produce breast milk. Sadness or crying will further diminish the chi and fluids. Fluids are also essential for lubrication during sex. See the recipes in appendix 5 for some wonderful soups for the postpartum period, like the nettle bone broth and kitchari. *The First Forty Days* is an amazing postpartum cookbook and resource that has over forty recipes and is a wonderful complement to the information and recipes shared here.

Community Stories:
Circe

....

Circe is a former professional snowboarder and an action-sports agent, in a male-dominated testosterone-driven industry. She is the only woman among ten male agents at her agency. Her teens and twenties were spent squeezing every ounce out of life. Traveling all over the world, partying, snowboarding, and surfing, she thoroughly enjoyed meeting important people and taking care of her high-profile clients. When she had her first baby at thirty-two, it was wintertime, which was high season for her clients. When her baby was five weeks old, she was on a plane headed for the Sundance Film Festival and the Winter X Games. Baby in the carrier, cell phone in one hand, diaper bag on the other shoulder, becoming a mother was not going to slow her down. She continued to build her stable of clients and was adored and admired for her commitment to mothering, bringing her baby with her to events so that she could continue nursing and parenting.

When Circe had her second baby at forty, she was back in action and on calls within four days. This time her recovery was not so smooth. She started to experience digestive issues, food allergies, eczema, and was eventually diagnosed with an autoimmune disorder. She embarked on a journey to heal her gut through diet and sleep, and was forced to slow down. The second birth pushed her over a threshold into energetic debt. You could say that she was a person with a tremendous amount of original life force and resiliency. She managed a demanding lifestyle of worldwide travel, big-money deals, and a high-profile clientele and still seemed to exert herself physically with little effort. However, without carving out time after either birth for full recovery, her body began to break down. She could no longer override this compounded health debt without intensive focus on rebuilding her whole system. It has taken a few years of intense focus on rebuilding her gut, as well as a deliberate slowing down to allow her to reach a new level of vitality.

It is also helpful to season food with spices that have warming properties, like ginger, black pepper, and cinnamon. Avoid cold foods like ice cream and iced water, which can transfer cold to the uterus and increase the energy needed for digestion, energy that a woman doesn't have to spare postpartum. Often in the West, in a desire to heal as fast as possible, women adopt their old strategies of what worked for getting into shape and regaining health, just as I did, without taking into account their new normal. We might choose juices, salads, and smoothies in an attempt to eat healthfully and lose the baby weight, but cold and raw foods are actually taxing for the system at this time and will deplete us further, when what we need is to nourish and rebuild blood and yin.

It is imperative that the mother be served regular meals with protein and warm broths to replenish fluids and to help form new blood and breast milk. Dietary fat in particular is a yin substance that is necessary for the production of breast milk. Doctors of Chinese medicine use all manner of plants, minerals, and animals in their herbal formulas. It is said that when bodily substance (blood, yin, and essence) is needed, sometimes only "flesh and blood" medicinal substances will suffice. That means that for some women, eating meat will be critical in order to get the iron and other minerals that they need.

And not to be a killjoy, but please take note: if you start dropping weight quickly or suddenly, keep in mind that your breastfeeding baby is probably drawing not from energy you have to spare but from your energy reserves, which is a recipe for depletion. Take care to eat three regular meals per day, with two nutritious snacks in between. Make sure your food choices have an adequate amount of healthy protein and fat. This will keep your blood-sugar levels steady and will help you rebuild your energy and have enough stores for your baby.

Mother Roasting in Chinese Medicine

Asian cultures take mother warming very seriously. Women are admonished to keep the abdomen and low back covered at all times in the months after having a baby. Young Chinese women suffer through their visiting mother-in-law's insistence that the windows stay closed, so no drafts may enter, while the stuffy apartment reeks of the day's herbs boiling in a pot on the stove. Women are encouraged to take herbal baths rather than showering to keep the head warm. Not everyone is happily compliant, but most are respectful of the ancient traditions passed down through the generations of women in their family.

In East Asian medicine, "mother roasting" can be literal: it refers specifically to an acupuncturist applying moxibustion to acupuncture points on the lower abdomen and low back. The yang energy of the moxa (mugwort floss) helps to seal the lower back and abdomen, protecting the mother from low back pain and prolapse (sinking of chi), and helps secure the kidney chi (preventing incontinence) and other lingering problems.

NOURISHING THROUGH AYURVEDIC TRADITION

Ayurveda is the ancient system of healing in India. Ayurveda is a sister science to yoga, both of which grew out of the school of thought in India called Sankhya philosophy. Translated, *ayurveda* means "the science of life," and provides a system of healing for the mind, body, and spirit that yoga seeks to harmonize. As asanas, or poses, are the yoga of the body, Ayurveda is the yoga of medicine.

Where Western medicine utilizes generalized treatment strategies for alleviating the symptoms of disease, Ayurveda addresses the root of illness and imbalance according to the unique constitution of the individual. It is practiced as a part of everyday life and considers conditions like the weather, the season, and the individual essence of a person in determining optimal healing choices. Those lifestyle choices range from what to eat and what spices or herbs to use, to the breathing and movement practices that best support a person's wellness.

Wellness is akin to wholeness. We make ourselves whole when we remember that we are made of the same elements found in nature and that our true nature is spirit. This planetary medicine honors the interdependence of everything—mineral, plant, animal, and human—and encourages us to tune in to the rhythms of nature and utilize her gifts for our healing.

Ayurveda understands that the mind and body are inextricably linked and have infinite influence over each other. It also understands that healing the one is healing the other. Like Chinese medicine, the goal of Ayurvedic medicine is not to simply get better when we are sick or even to prevent illness from occurring in the first place, although they both do these effectively. The aim is for each person to live in such exquisite harmony that she can live her life's purpose to her fullest potential and be in alignment with life force itself.

There is a saying in Ayurveda: You aren't what you eat but rather what you digest and assimilate. In Ayurvedic medicine, our ability to digest food, thoughts, feelings, experiences, and everything else in our environment determines the quality of our health and well-being. According to this tradition, if we are digesting, assimilating, and eliminating well, we will be happy. When we are able to digest everything we take in through our senses, including our emotions and life experiences, then our digestive fire, *agni*, can adequately sort out what we need to assimilate and convert into building material from what we need to eliminate.

What Is Agni?

Let's just take a moment to understand the important role of agni, or digestive fire. Agni dwells in every cell of the body, and converts food into different kinds of tissue. There are seven different kinds of vital tissues (*dhatus*): plasma, blood, muscle, fat, bone, the tissues of the nervous system, and reproductive tissues. They are nourished in succession. If one tissue is formed poorly, the following tissue that it is built upon cannot be nourished properly.

The most important tissue to nourish postpartum is *rasa*. Rasa, meaning "juice" or "taste," forms our lymph and the plasma part of our blood. It is the basis of all other tissue formation and detoxification. Postpartum, a woman's rasa is most often decreased due to the loss of fluid from the body after pregnancy and breastfeeding. Factors that further deplete rasa are lifestyle choices that also increase *vata*, which will be explained later in this chapter.

Secondary tissues (*upadhatu*) are produced when the primary tissues are well nourished and substantial. For example, the upadhatus of rasa are breast milk and menstrual blood. If rasa is depleted, a new mother may have a low milk supply.

Agni is the force that determines what becomes primary tissues (dhatu), what becomes secondary tissue (upadhatu), and what becomes waste (*mala*). A woman needs to both eat and digest enough tissue-building food so that there is substance enough to form breast milk without having to leech from her own energy stores and decrease her own vital tissues. The body will take what it needs to make the breast milk, but if a woman isn't sufficiently fortified, she will be borrowing from her own tissues to do so. Agni must also be kept strong and regular to keep toxicity from blocking the channels of tissue formation.

Thus, the food we eat, when digested well, literally becomes the sweet, nourishing breast milk we feed our babies, and contributes to the overall development of *ojas*, which is akin to the baby's immune system.

What Is Ojas?

After plasma, blood, muscle, fat, bone, the tissues of the nervous system, and the tissues of the reproductive system (*shukra*) are formed, an eighth tissue develops: ojas. Ojas contains our life energy, provides stability to the body and mind, and strengthens the immune system.

Strengthening Agni and Revitalizing Ojas

In the postpartum period, new moms are most susceptible to weakened agni and low ojas. Ayurvedic medicine focuses on strengthening and revitalizing both agni and ojas through simple but important practices involving the proper intake of food. Eating at regular times, eating while sitting down, and eating food that is easy to digest are the simplest ways to begin to rekindle agni. When digestion is easy, a woman's body can focus only on healing and rebuilding instead of the work of digesting. For this reason, as in Chinese medicine, special care is taken with postpartum food preparation and presentation.

A woman can rebuild her ojas during her fourth trimester through eating certain foods, such as dates, milk, ghee, and sesame; taking herbs such as ashwaganda, shatavari, and brahmi; taking time to rest her body and mind and bond with her baby; spending time in nature; meditating and keeping her rasa nourished through sweet demulcent teas (licorice or fennel); ample fluid intake through bone broth, soups, and stews; and plenty of warm-oil massage.

Food is prepared with specific herbs that aid in digestion, as food and herbs are the material by which ojas can be rebuilt and potentiated. Rest, love, and compassion also contribute to ojas. In keeping with the postpartum practice of staying slow, a new mom can begin to rebuild her ojas by filling up on quiet, simple moments like gazing into her newborn's eyes, becoming aware of her own breath while feeding her baby, and limiting the use of unnecessary time on screens, such as the computer or phone. In Chinese medicine, women are told to rest their eyes, in particular in the months following childbirth, as the eyes are related to the amount of blood a woman has. Resting one's eyes is important to not tax the blood in the liver, both the organ and meridian, which is already deficient in postpartum women. Certainly some time checking-in on social media, responding to e-mails, or doing online shopping can be practical and even restorative, but excessive time on screens depletes life force, and screen gazing should ideally be minimized during this sacred time. Conversely, prayer and meditation, which clarify the mind, get us closer to our hearts and usher us into contact with the divine.

Understanding the Three Doshas: Vata, Pitta, and Kapha

Ayurveda holds that everything in the material world is made of a combination of five elements of nature—earth, water, fire, air, and ether. The presence, or absence, of each element and their combination and proportion determines the form of an object. When combined in human beings, the elements are grouped into three categories called *doshas*, or constitutions. Each of us has a combination of the elements that shifts throughout our lives depending on our environment and lifestyle, but we enter the world with both a divine and genetic predisposition that makes one or two of the doshas more dominant. The three doshas are *vata*, *pitta*, and *kapha*, and there are infinite possibilities for their expression.

Vata, directly translated as "wind," consists of air and ether and governs all movement in the body and mind. Vata is responsible for

Cooking Postpartum

I believe that having someone in your home cooking for you, like a postpartum doula or a loving friend or family member, establishes a rhythm that is soothing for everyone. You can't rush how fast the food cooks (unless you microwave it, which I don't advocate). There is something primary and basic about tending to our relationship to this most basic element of the earth, respecting the time it takes to select, prepare, and cook food. Each pot on the stove cooks in its own time. A mother can relax when she knows she will have enough food and be fed well. This is food that is lovingly prepared, delicious, and nourishing for you and your family. Then, baby can relax because mom is relaxed. Both Ayurveda and Chinese medicine emphasize that new moms eat food that is made fresh each day for optimal nutrition.

And, by the way, takeout and frozen foods have their place as well! I would rather you, as a new mom, have something to eat than go without food at all. If the majority of meals are warm, home-cooked, balanced, and easily digestible, a little takeout or leftovers won't hurt. This isn't about perfection—it is about attention!

elimination, muscular movements, sensory input to the brain, the nervous system, and the circulation of nutrients in all cellular tissue. Vata is the most important of the doshas, because when vata is out of balance, it will often push the other doshas out of balance.

Pitta is derived from the elements of fire and water and rules digestion and metabolism.

Kapha is produced by the combination of the elements earth and water and provides structure and stability to the body, as well as lubrication and strength.

Your Dosha Type

Vata types move quickly and are typically thin. They don't love cold weather and tend to have dry hair and dry skin. Even their minds move quickly; they are fast learners. Vata types tend toward anxiety. They experience light and fitful sleep.

Pitta-dominant people have a muscular build and, when out of balance, can have an impatient, fiery disposition. Pittas have good digestion and don't like to miss meals. They don't like hot and dry weather. They are known for their sharp intellect, good memory, and leadership qualities. Pittas usually sleep well and wake up rested.

Kapha types are known for their steadiness and reliability. They have softer, rounder bodies that have a tendency toward weight gain. You can recognize kaphas by their large, doe-like eyes and pale skin. They sleep a lot and can skip meals, as their digestion is slow. Where the quick vata types tend toward anxiety, slow kapha types tend toward depression. People with kapha constitutions have the most energy, though it may not appear so on the surface. They are slow burners, and rarely burn out.

Getting into your specific type, and most of us are a combination, is beyond the scope of this book. The most important thing to understand about the doshas for our purposes is that all women will experience a vata imbalance in the postpartum period. During labor and childbirth, vata, in the form of the downward wind (*apana vayu*), is the force that helps to bring the baby down the birth canal and out through the vagina. Even if a woman gives birth through a cesarean section, she experiences an increase in vata.

After the baby is born and the womb is empty, vata remains present in the form of space. If a woman already has a vata constitution, then the vata imbalance will be exaggerated. Regardless, a vata imbalance can leave a woman scattered and off-center, with a vulnerability to cold and dryness. Ayurvedic practice recommends that, during the sacred window, new mothers take specific care to balance vata aggravation by balancing the qualities of vata—cold, light, mobile, dry, and rough—with their opposites—hot, heavy, static, moist, and smooth. The three main avenues to move the system back toward balance and wholeness are warmth, oils, and moisture.

Eat Your Placenta?

The use of placenta for postpartum healing is a convergence of the back-to-the-land movement and the importation and interpretation of traditional Chinese medicine to the United States. The ethos of the back-to-the-land movement was for humans to mirror nature: since animals eat their own placentas, we should too. Raven Lang, a homebirth midwife in the early 1960s, would prepare a placenta stew after the birth that would be eaten communally. In the 1980s, when her practice became more urban, she began making placenta capsules which were easier for many women to ingest.

The effects of placenta consumption are not yet scientifically known. Many women report more stable moods, less weepiness, and an easier recovery after birth. Fortunately, there are no known negative effects. Most likely a placenta pill has the combination of a homeopathic and placebo effect. If your body needs the hormones, then it will use them, if not, they'll be eliminated. Perhaps we can also leave a little room for the magic of ritual acknowledgment and embracing our animal self.

Mother Warming

Ayurvedic attention to warmth in the postpartum period dovetails with Chinese medicine's and other traditional cultures worldwide. Warmth in both the external environment and what we put in our bodies will help counteract the tendency for elemental cold to arise after childbirth. As mentioned above, in some East African countries, women sit over a scalding-hot steam pot after giving birth in order to seal the vaginal opening and protect from wind and cold entering—a far cry from perineal ice packs that are so often recommended in American hospitals. In rural Mexico, new mothers are cared for in a "closing of the bones" ceremony, a four-part ritual that includes being in a sweat-lodge-like enclosure and drenched with very hot herbal water. Then the mother is mummy-wrapped to seal in the warmth and allow her to continue to sweat and detoxify.

In many cultures and traditions, ranging across Malaysia, Korea, Japan, Mexico, and Brazil, women are encouraged to stay bundled up. Belly-binding traditions not only protect and nudge the organs back into place, but also provide the mother with a sense of warmth and comfort, alleviating the feeling of emptiness. Being tightly wrapped allows a woman to feel the contours of her own body, providing a feeling of containment. A new mom is encouraged to wear layers of warm clothes and keep her feet warm. Herbal baths are drawn so the new mom can soak, and she is encouraged to stay in the bathroom until completely dressed.

Ways that you can implement mother warming at home include, but are not limited to,

- Drawing and taking herbal baths with fresh or dried herbs such as rosemary, chamomile, comfrey, ginger, eucalyptus, lime, lemongrass, and lavender, and then wrapping yourself in a warm robe and wearing socks afterward.
- Using a warm-water bottle on your low belly and lower back. Make sure that you have a cloth or towel between the water bottle and your skin, so you don't burn yourself. (For convenience,

you can use a heating pad, but be sure to get the kind that turns off automatically and won't burn you, so if you fall asleep, you'll still be safe.)

- Staying hydrated with warm herbal teas, rather than cold drinks.
- Trying belly binding. You can use a garment designed to give this support, like the AB tank from Bellies, Inc. Traditional belly-binding techniques are best learned from a postpartum doula. A doula can also teach one of your family members or friends how to wrap you. It is possible to wrap yourself. You can read the instructions on belly wrapping or even watch videos on YouTube to guide you through the process. More details and instructions on belly binding can be found in chapter 7.

Vaginal Steaming

So you thought you'd heard of everything. So did I. Enter vagina steaming, otherwise known as a *vajacial*, or "the other facial." Before you dismiss it as the latest fad, it turns out that women around the world have been giving themselves vagina steams with everything from goat's milk to turmeric to mugwort for ages. In countries from South Korea to Eritrea to Suriname, women routinely use vaginal steaming for gynecological health. If we go back a generation, in almost every corner of the world, we can find a tradition of vaginal steaming. Most people have heard of sitz baths—perineal soaks with herbs or Epsom salts, which I also recommend—but steaming is different in its ability to penetrate more deeply into the reproductive organs. The herbs used in the steam are absorbed through the porous mucosal tissue, and not just reproductive organs are affected—women report less swelling in the legs, relief for tender breasts, as well as less painful and more regular periods.

There are many potential benefits to vaginal steaming postpartum, including warming the body, healing the placental site, and aiding in clearing out any residue in the uterus. The steam creates warmth from the inside out, which is both therapeutic and deeply relaxing.

Heat also improves circulation of blood, lymph, and chi, which, together with medicinal herbs that have antiseptic and antibiotic properties, helps to clear out stagnation.

Stitches are notoriously hard to clean, but steaming with antiseptic herbs easily cleans the tissues without friction. Additionally, the steam helps organs return to their optimal positions. Women have reported that steams assist with prolapses, both soon after birth or even months to years later. Imagine a pot with a lid on it and how the steam is powerful enough to push the top up, so it teeters around with boiling water below. Similarly, when the steam enters a woman's body, the organs are encouraged upward. Keli Garza, known as the "Steamy Chick," is the world's leading expert on vaginal steaming and its uses all over the world. She herself steamed every day for thirty days postpartum starting two weeks after the birth, as part of her care regimen, which helped her bleed for less time, heal completely, and be ready to return to intimacy.

After a vaginal delivery, wait to steam until you are not bleeding heavily. If you are bleeding trace amounts, it is not only okay, but it is also helpful to steam to help your body clear out the residue from your uterus faster. Obviously if you are hemorrhaging, you need medical help, not steaming! If you have had a cesarean, steaming is still necessary and helpful: just wait six weeks and until the stitches are completely healed.

To do a vaginal steam, you will need a steam chair. There are videos on YouTube that show you how to rig your toilet for vaginal steaming, but the safest way is to use a chair that is designed especially for steaming, so your sensitive vulva is the right distance from the pot of steaming herbs.

I believe that this daily experience with our own vaginas postpartum could be one step toward reclamation of our bodies. I think vaginal steaming is a total game changer for women's early postpartum sexual encounters. Instead of feeling hesitant and afraid, women could return to sex with more confidence and self-knowledge.

Oil Is Love

The Sanskrit word for oil is *sneha*, which also means "love." Because out-of-balance vata tends toward dryness, new moms are encouraged to oil their bodies through food and massage. The heavy, soft, and smooth qualities of oil help to soothe the light, hard, and rough qualities that vata provokes. Eating healthy fats in the form of at least a tablespoon of grass-fed ghee, butter, or coconut oil with each meal is recommended for new moms, and even more when constipation and dryness are present. The oils nourish your tissues and help to strengthen your nervous system. If you are used to a low-fat diet, this tablespoon of fat with each meal probably seems like way too much. Don't worry: not all fats make you fat. Ghee, butter, and coconut oil are soothing and will contribute to the healing of your tissues, and transferred through breast milk, they will also contribute to your baby's brain development.

Another way to oil your body is through massage. Touch is a huge part of an Ayurvedic approach to postpartum healing. Abhyanga, or oil massage, is recommended for the first forty-two days. Yes, daily massage! Doesn't that sound like heaven? Indians and Nepalese consider daily massage in postpartum a necessity, not a luxury. Soothing, rhythmic massage helps to restore the nervous system and rid the body of toxins accumulated during pregnancy. During a time when things can be disorienting and many women feel overwhelmed, frequent massage can help you remain calm, centered, and grounded. Sesame, almond, coconut, and apricot oils are known to calm vata and can be good massage oils.

If you don't have someone to massage you, treat yourself to a self-massage. Standing in a warm bathroom or sitting on a towel you don't care much about, cover yourself generously with your chosen oil. Be sure to warm it up by running the bottle under hot water first or placing it in a bowl of hot water for a few minutes prior to beginning your massage. Start at the center of your body and move outward, to the limbs. Use long, gentle, loving strokes, and circles at your joints.

Massage your abdomen in a clockwise motion that follows the direction of your intestines. Don't miss your scalp. After about fifteen minutes, enjoy a warm bath or shower. Make sure to rinse your feet first, so you don't slip. Designate a towel to be your post-massage towel, because eventually it will get ruined from all the oil. Take care when washing these towels. You will want to add some vinegar and baking soda to the hot water once the washing machine is full. Hang drying the oil-soaked towel is best because in high heat, the oil can become flammable.

How to Hydrate

The third vata-calming technique is moisture. Moisture is the most straightforward. Hydrate well by drinking water, teas, and liquid-y soups. Avoid dehydration by eliminating caffeine, alcohol, and soft drinks. If your baby was born in the summer, boil a quart of water with two tablespoons each of cumin seeds, coriander seeds, and fennel seeds (CCF); strain, let cool, and sip throughout the day. This CCF tea will help restore your digestive fires without overheating your body. Enjoy CCF tea served hot in the winter. Avoid iced drinks throughout all the seasons, so as not to dampen or chill your digestive organs. If all you remember is to keep yourself warm, hydrated, and sufficiently oiled, this will be a big step forward in your postpartum care.

Both Ayurveda and Chinese medicine take us back to the wisdom of the land, reminding us that certain foods only grow at certain times of the year, and the wisdom of the life cycle, reminding us that certain foods are most appropriate for certain moments in our lives. No matter how well a woman has cared for herself, birth requires recovery. The more peaceful and thorough the recovery, the quicker the return to total health.

While most of us view this kind of care as a luxury, we should recategorize it as necessity. Many women wouldn't think of giving birth without the support of a doula because evidence shows that labor with doula support is shorter and has fewer interventions. And yet, fifteen

The Sacred Window School

Ysha Oakes, a great innovator and advocate for women, created the profession of "Ayudoulas" in the United States and established the Sacred Window School. She trained postpartum doulas in Ayurvedic cooking and massage as well as the spiritual and yogic understanding of the passage into motherhood. She had studied and been trained by the Maharishi Mahesh, of Beatles fame, in his Mother and Baby Program that established this model of six weeks of total care for mother and baby.

Ysha Oakes reported that in a small sample of thirty-five participants in the Mother and Baby Program none of the women experienced depression, at a time when one in seven women was being diagnosed with depression. Sonya Bastow, an Ayudoula in Boulder, Colorado, reported that in thirteen years of supporting hundreds of families postpartum, she could count on one hand the number of women who experienced baby blues or postpartum depression while working with her. None of the mothers whom she cared for between three and six days a week for six weeks experienced depression! She also shared that many moms hired her after having their second baby and remarked that it was a totally different experience. They reported they were not as weepy as they were after they had their first baby, that it was a relief to have someone else in the house with them during the day, and that they felt like everything was going to be okay.

years ago, no one knew what the word *doula* meant. Today doulas are hired by hospitals, and many men and women understand their role.

A study published in the British journal *Birth* found that only 4.7 percent of women using doulas had preterm births, and 20.4 percent had cesarean deliveries, compared with respective figures of 6.3 percent and 34.2 percent for those who did not work with a doula. Other studies cited in "Support for Women in Childbirth" in *Cochrane Database of Systematic Reviews* have shown that having a doula as part of the birth team decreases the length of labor by 25 percent, the use of pitocin by 40 percent, and requests for an epidural by 60 percent.

We are still waking up to the importance of the postpartum period. Currently, there is no quantitative research concerning how helpful a postpartum doula is to a woman's short- and long-term recovery from birth. But ask any woman who has invested in a postpartum doula, and she will tell you it was the best investment she ever made. Having the presence of a wise woman who comes to offer loving touch, prepare nutritious food, draw herbal baths, and easily facilitate all of these natural healing techniques is priceless.

But even without hiring professional help, it's important to realize that you don't have to be an expert in Chinese or Ayurvedic medicine to implement some of the simple principles to enhance your postpartum healing. Nourishing yin qualities and calming vata are the most important principles to remember. You can do both of these by prioritizing rest, eating nourishing foods, and keeping yourself warm, all of which are investments in your long-term health and strength.

SUMMARY

- Chinese and Ayurvedic medicine agree that a woman's life force is depleted in the birth process and needs to be tended to and strengthened in the postpartum period so that she can fully recover and return to robust health.
- Post-birth women are often yin and blood deficient. Food and warming practices will help to rebuild blood and yin so that women have enough fluids.
- All women will experience a vata imbalance postpartum. The three ways to calm vata are oil, heat, and hydration.

Reflections

- What is one thing you can do right now to nourish yin?
- Consider the different Chinese fluids and if you may see a pattern in your life of being particularly low or high in any of them.
- Read the descriptions of the different doshas. Can you identify what your predominant dosha is? Do you already have a tendency toward vata imbalance? If so, what practices can you start now to help you to balance vata?

Practices

- Wear warm clothes, especially socks.
- Keep your abdomen, low back, nape of neck, and feet covered.
- Swaddle in warm blankets.
- Take sitz baths.
- Try vaginal steaming.
- Drink herbal teas.
- Keep your environment warm.
- Do not sit around with wet hair.
- Avoid drafts, fans, and sleeping by an open window.
- Rest your eyes and limit screen time.
- Avoid lifting anything heavy.
- Avoid strong emotions, especially anger.
- Avoid cold raw foods.
- Eat black sesame seeds, walnuts, greens, beets, chicken, eggs, beef, seaweed, miso, and fish if cooked with ginger and rice wine.
- Cook with warming herbs (black pepper, ginger, cinnamon, and cardamom).
- Use moxibustion (artmesia argyi/mugwort) to warm the low belly from the pubic bone to the navel for five to ten minutes, four to five days after the birth.

rebuilding your body

Miraculously, and often disconcertingly, our bodies continue to change shape, with our weight shifting and redistributing after birth. Our breasts and bellies are in continual flux as milk descends. Our organs shrink and shift to find their optimal homes now that a baby is no longer present. Every glance in the mirror shows previously unknown and unfamiliar proportions.

Not to sound like a broken record, but rebuilding your body begins with—you guessed it—rest. There is no easy way to say it: even though giving birth is a natural event, and women have been doing it for centuries, it takes a toll on your body. Birth requires a recovery period. It's inaccurate to think that you can just go on with your daily life and normal activities as if you haven't just spent ten months pregnant and gone through a major bodily event.

During pregnancy, your uterus was stretched to more than five times its normal size. If your baby came out vaginally, your cervix and vaginal canal shape-shifted to open a pathway for your baby, your organs were squeezed to the sides, and the perineal skin stretched taut. It's not an everyday event that your body is used to. If your baby was born via cesarean section, you had at least four layers—skin, connective tissue, muscle, and organ—cut through. If you had an anesthetic during birth, it takes time to leave your system. Also, all women experience a dramatic flood of surging and dropping and rebalancing of hormones after giving birth.

The recovery period is different for every woman and can be influenced by factors as concrete as how long your gestation was, how long your labor was, what happened during the birth, how many pregnancies you have experienced (including miscarriages and abortions), how much sleep you are getting, and factors as seemingly unrelated as how nurtured you feel, how supportive your partner is if you have one, and when you have to go back to work.

But across the board, midwives agree that—irrespective of all those individual considerations—all women should spend the first fifteen days after giving birth in total repose. The saying goes: five days in the bed, five days on the bed, and five days around the bed.

That's fifteen days barely leaving your room, keeping your legs closed, and minimizing your movements. This rest allows for restoration at the deepest level. Your pelvic fibers can reknit themselves and heal any tears or "skid marks," skin scrapes that don't require stitches but are still painful. The psyche has time to integrate the experience without additional input. The whole physical body enjoys stillness, so the internal organs can settle and recalibrate.

During those first fifteen days, an appropriate way to reconnect with your body is through gentle breathing. You'll want to return to the breath for length. Gentle breathing will allow you to connect to your core and can help balance your nervous system. Twice a day, for at least two minutes, close your eyes and focus on the movement of your breath in your chest, ribs, belly, and pelvis. If you have any discomfort during deep breathing, then it isn't time yet. If you had a cesarean and feel the scar or adhesion pulling, wait just a few more days and start again. You don't need to do any restorative pelvic-floor work yet. Just allow the natural intelligence of your body to prove itself in its own time. These four minutes will also establish a habit of coming back to a connection with your body, your self, and the present moment every day. Ideally this is done in a position called constructive rest (see fig. 11), which requires the least effort to maintain. Lie down on your back, with your feet flat on the floor and a bit wider than your hips. Let your knees fall together and rest against each other.

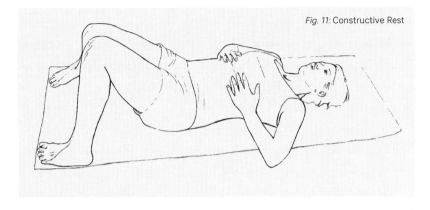

Fig. 11: Constructive Rest

REBUILD YOUR CORE

Training the core is the most important part of the birth-recovery process, and, when attended to, it is the key to feeling really vibrant and strong again. But what exactly is your core? We hear about it all the time and typically think of it in regard to our abs and doing "core work." But working the core is more than just doing crunches. The core is made up of four main muscle groups—the pelvic floor, breathing diaphragm, transversus abdominis, and multifidi. Janet Hulme, author of the *Pelvic Rotator Cuff* and a pelvic-health physical therapist, calls these muscles the "Core Four." These muscle groups are critical for posture and organ support. When they are well balanced, we hardly notice them, especially since they are layered, and many of them are groups of small muscles. They are not like pectoral muscles or biceps that bulge when we engage them, making it obvious what happens when they are activated. They are stabilizers that help create balance. All of the common complaints that new moms have about back pain, neck and shoulder pain, sacroiliac discomfort, and joint pain can be traced back to some element of dysfunction in the core or too much load on an already stressed region of the core.

The pelvic floor is an interconnected and multitiered team of muscles that surrounds the lower body openings and also creates a buoyant shelf for the bladder, uterus, and rectum. These muscles form a tether to the base of the spine.

The breathing diaphragm is a large and relatively thin sheath of muscle that attaches all the way around the rib basket. It drops when we inhale, like an inverted umbrella, and rises as we exhale, returning to the normal umbrella shape.

The transversus abdominis, or transverse abdominal muscle, is known as the TA or corset muscle. It is deeper than the rectus abdominis, which are the six-pack muscles, and wraps from the spine all the way around to the front of the body. Baby wraps that you wear mirror what these muscles do.

The multifidi are a series of small muscles that attach one vertebra to another along the spine and allow for tiny postural adjustments, balance corrections, and uprightness.

All four of these muscle groups have to be able to fire and coordinate for complete core engagement. After having a baby, many women need to remind themselves to engage their cores first, before beginning exertion. If you resume heavier exercise too early, without first making sure that the core is active first, there will be undue pressure on other body parts, requiring compensations. If one part of the body isn't doing its job, another will usually step in, but it may cause discomfort because it'll put you out of alignment. Mothering requires a lot of awkward movements—picking up the baby, putting in car seats and carrying them, twisting around to see how the baby is doing, and breastfeeding. To be able to do these movements without hurting yourself, there has to be support from the inside.

Muscles are intrinsic or extrinsic. *Extrinsic muscles* are the larger muscle groups, many of which we can see and with names most of us are familiar with, for example, quads, biceps, and trapezius. These bigger muscles are in charge of big movements. *Intrinsic muscles* are smaller and closer to the skeleton. They are related to our reflexes and help to initiate movement as well as coordinate balance.

According to the Rolf Method of Structural Integration, movement in a healthy body is balanced between the intrinsic and extrinsic muscle systems. Ideally, they work together in a coordinated fashion. After giving birth, the intrinsic muscles are compromised and take some time to return to function. Often, the extrinsic muscles are working extra hard to maintain balance in the structure. More specifically, because the pelvic-floor muscles are overstretched and weak, the outer hip muscles and rotators grip to stabilize the pelvis. Because the stomach muscles are loose and weak, the muscles in the lower back and at the pelvic rim tighten to brace the spine.

As all levels of our being are connected, our core also contributes to feeling stable, secure, and at home in the world and in our bodies. When the core is weak, many women feel untethered, scattered, and indecisive as well as fearful. When the core is overly tight, women may feel hard, stuck, and a numbness that makes it difficult to contact deep feelings. When the core is firm and stable, a woman will feel as if she has access to her inner world and an inner compass that will help guide her decisions and actions.

Wrapping Your Belly
About three to seven days after your baby is born, you may want to wrap your belly to help your organs return to their optimal positions, to give your lower back a little extra support, and to encourage your abdominal muscles to return closer to each other. Belly wrapping might seem trendy, but for hundreds of years in Malaysia, Indonesia, Nepal, India, and Taiwan, postnatal care has included belly wrapping and belly binding. Also remember that, from the perspective of Ayurveda and Chinese medicine, belly wrapping provides less opportunity for cold or wind to enter the body. There are also some modern versions of belly wraps that are less specific, more practical, and still effective.

To support healthy abdominal and pelvic recovery, you want to make sure that the wrap or band you are using doesn't just squeeze your waist; if you cinch your waist tightly without also supporting your pelvis, you could place downward pressure on your pelvic floor, which can contribute to or exacerbate chronically weakened tissues and issues, such as prolapse. An ideal wrap is secured from the bottom up and lifts your organs and belly, while bringing them closer to your midline.

In Chinese medicine, the meridian that runs from the perineum up the midline of the body to the face is called *ren mai*, which is translated as the conception vessel, or CV. The point CV 1 is cut if there is an episiotomy; it is also affected by tearing. CV 4 is disrupted by cesarean surgery. Wrapping the belly can protect this channel, which is the meridian most closely related to mothering and the mother archetype.

In sum, belly wrapping can help:

- heal or prevent a diastasis (separation of the abdominal walls);
- improve your posture and prevent lower back pain and sacroiliac pain;
- increase warmth (calming vata); and
- help your pelvic ligaments gel back together and not stretch further.

How to Belly Wrap

There are belly-wrapping practices in cultures from India to Taiwan, and each has its own unique twist. What they have in common are the above intentions to keep women protected from wind and cold, and to help prevent lower back pain by providing upright support for the organs and the core.

The Malaysian tradition of belly binding utilizes a cloth called a *bengkung*. For ease of understanding, I am going to call this cloth a *belt*. This belt is at least twenty-six feet in length—and can be as long as forty feet if you are tall or have a longer torso—and about six to eight inches in width. With such a long piece of cloth, wrapping is easier and more efficient when the belt is rolled. Some people put the long end in a basket or plastic bag so they can kick it around as they wrap. I recommend storing the belt already rolled, so it is easy to handle and ready for use.

Below are basic, step-by-step instructions for bengkung-style belly wrapping when doing it by yourself. Wear a tank top so that you don't have to wash the cloth often and the twists don't pinch your skin.

1. Start standing up in front of a full-length mirror. Unroll the belt until you have a piece of cloth the same length as your torso measuring from your pubic bone to your forehead. That piece is called the tail. Place the end of it over your shoulder or in between your teeth.

2. Start at your midline. Unroll the belt and wrap the width of the belt around your hips, behind your back, and over to the other side. (Although this is called belly binding, you want to wrap your hips to begin with and move upward to the belly.)

3. Now cinch it tight as you wrap the tail against the long end for one full turn, so the end is positioned how it began and the still-to-be-unrolled belt is close to the body again. Some people put the long-rolled end in a basket and kick it around them as they wrap. The tail goes back up over your shoulder. Eventually you want a total of ten to fourteen twists.

4. The widths of the fabric overlap and you will have to fan open the width each time you take the fabric around your waist or hips.

5. Pull slightly to adjust tension, and wrap again from the other side back around the back until the roll and the end meet again at the midline. Keep holding the tail in front. You want the twists to line up so using a mirror will help you verify that.

6. Adjust tension accordingly and keep wrapping, twisting the two cloths at the midline each time.

7. At the top, tie a knot and tuck in the ends.

The bengkung belly wrapping generally follows a belly massage with herbs like ginger, clove, fennel, and lemongrass to warm your abdomen, lower back, and breasts. While it is wonderful to receive this herbal massage from a bodyworker, and I highly recommend you do receive skilled bodywork if you can, you can also massage yourself with one or a combination of these herbs prior to wrapping yourself.

Women are encouraged to wear their wrap for at least six hours and up to the whole day, but not sleeping in it, for the first four to six weeks after birth. The Malaysians and Indonesians, like most Asian cultures, observe a forty- to forty-eight-day confinement period, where elder female family members take care of the new mother. A postpartum doula can assist your partner or a trusted friend in teaching you how to wrap, if you are not getting the hang of it. There are also a few short videos on the Internet that you can watch until you get the hang of it. The first couple times are awkward, but after that it will take you between five and ten minutes.

Take care if your wrists are sensitive, so they are not strained while pulling the belt to create the right amount of tension. (Wrists are extra sensitive postpartum because of the movements required for breastfeeding and carrying babies and because the softer ligaments create unstable joints.) Between day three and day ten after giving birth, when the heavy bleeding has stopped, begin wrapping. You'll have to experiment to figure out how tightly to wrap yourself. When being wrapped, most women are surprised at how tight the wrap is, but also at how good it feels. If these wrapping techniques seem too complicated, many women will opt for a ready-made one-piece option. I recommend the AB wrap from Bellies, Inc. that is easy-to-use, comfortable, and washable.

Belly binding isn't a miracle cure to remove excess weight, but it can assist your body in returning to its prepregnancy shape, energy, and vitality. Some women worry that providing extra support will make their belly muscles weak. Remember that the wrapping is not just for muscular buttressing, but also for energetic and psychological reinforcement. Your entire being is recovering and needs support. Ysha Oakes of the Sacred Window Ayudoula healing school shared that belly wrapping is like being hugged at a time when there is stretched tissue and empty space inside. The body is able to work so much better, without as much slip and slide on the connections. Belly wrapping can help tissue rejuvenation, bowel function, and digestion. Even hormones and mood will be supported.

REBUILDING YOUR STRENGTH

After those first fifteen days, gentle movement together with breathing will build a strong base for lasting recovery and health. Attending to the core and to the intrinsic muscles will create a foundation that will allow you to return to training and to be able to use your extrinsic muscles without hurting yourself.

During this time, it is quality, not quantity that counts. Unlike the common wisdom that suggests we do Kegels at every phone ring and stoplight, it's not necessary to be on-call all day long for a pelvic-floor squeeze. Consistency, however, is important. It's better to do one exercise well for five minutes a day than to do a thirty-minute practice or an hour-and-a-half workout once a week. A little goes a long way when reactivating and training intrinsic muscles. If, at any time, you notice that you start to bleed more or that you are in pain after the movements—other than muscle soreness—then you probably overdid it.

And remember this is not the time to try to go to your limit and extend your flexibility. Your ligaments are still recovering, so it may feel like your muscles are being stretched while exercising, but at this time that "stretch" is actually the material that is keeping your bones together becoming more taffy-like—not what we want in the already fluid days of postpartum.

Yoga

These days, yoga is presented as a cure-all—good for everything, even doctors recommend it! But your practice needs to be the right yoga for the right time. Yoga that emphasizes leg strengthening, core engagement, or upper back opening is great during this time of recovery. Hip openers are not. Many women write to me confused about why their back or pelvis is hurting them after their yoga practice. This discomfort is often because they are using their prenatal yoga sequence as a template for what to do after they have a baby. The aims of prenatal yoga are the exact opposite of the aims for postpartum practice. In prenatal yoga, we emphasize opening and expanding the pelvis and encouraging downward action, making space for the baby. Our postpartum movement should help our bones and ligaments gel back together, lift everything back up, and nourish the cores of our bodies.

The postpartum time is an opportunity to expand our ideas of yoga practice. Yoga is about listening to and adapting to the needs of our bodies at a given moment. The following movement menu includes poses that help seal the pelvis, lengthen the spine, and relieve upper and lower back pain. The suggested poses are safe even if you have experienced a birth injury or diastasis.

WEEK-BY-WEEK MOVEMENT MENU

Every movement described here begins with the breath. Finish your exhalations to the very end, so you feel your low belly tone and quicken. Finishing your exhalation may be more of an image than an actual movement, but that is why we are doing it—to wake up these low belly muscles. Build your strengthening routine with each week, adding the new exercises that are listed to the ones you did each week before.

For all of the exercises that reference a ball, the prop used is a soft 6-inch diameter ball, but you can also use a 4x6x9-inch yoga block or a tightly rolled regular-sized bath towel. A ball would be the most useful and comfortable choice for the leg rotations.

Week One

Start with the Dynamic Wall Bridge.

DYNAMIC WALL BRIDGE WITH FEET ON THE WALL, USING A BALL

1. Lie down on your back, with your pelvis about sixteen inches away from the wall.
2. Place a ball between your mid thighs, lightly squeezing the ball as you slowly lift your hips up, articulating your spine (see fig. 12).
3. With your knees at a ninety-degree angle, press your feet into the wall and isometrically pull your heels down to activate your hamstrings and gluteus muscles as you roll up and down through your spine (see fig. 13). This should feel like some work in your inner legs as well as a massage along your spine and back muscles.
4. Exhale as you lift your hips up, and inhale as you lower your hips.
5. Repeat this five to ten times.

Note: The ball between your legs is so that you can feel a connection between your inner thighs and lower belly. Imagine that you are trying to pull the block in toward your pelvis, as well as squeezing it. As you do so, feel the band of muscles called the transversus abdominis that are like a low-slung seat belt. Feel the breath movement and low-slung activation as the initiator of movement. If you can't feel it, don't worry; the actions themselves can help wake the muscles up.

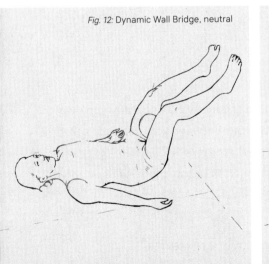

Fig. 12: Dynamic Wall Bridge, neutral

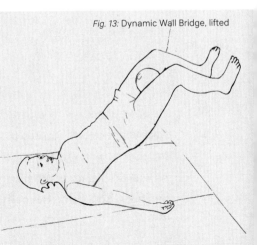

Fig. 13: Dynamic Wall Bridge, lifted

Week Two

Add the Charlie Chaplin/Pigeon Toes, and Floor Bridge.

CHARLIE CHAPLIN/PIGEON TOES

1. On your back, with your pelvis about one-and-a-half feet from the wall, extend your legs up the wall.

2. With a ball between your mid thighs, rotate your thighbones out, so your toes point away from each other, à la Charlie Chaplin (see fig. 14).

3. Then rotate your thighbones inward, so your toes are pointing inward, or pigeon-toed (see fig. 15). Maintain the squeeze of the ball.

4. Rotate out on the exhale; then, inhale and return your legs to neutral with feet parallel.

5. On your next exhale, rotate your legs inward, and inhale return to neutral.

6. Do three to five full sets of leg rotations.

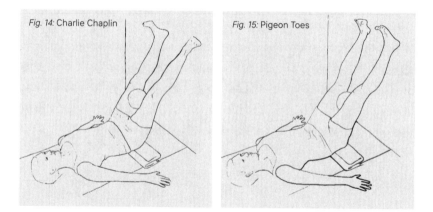

Fig. 14: Charlie Chaplin

Fig. 15: Pigeon Toes

FLOOR BRIDGE

1. Lie on your back with your feet hip distance apart, about a foot away from your bottom. You can place a ball between your mid thighs (see fig. 16).

2. As you exhale, lift your tailbone up, then pelvis, then low back, then mid back, squeezing the ball (see fig. 17).

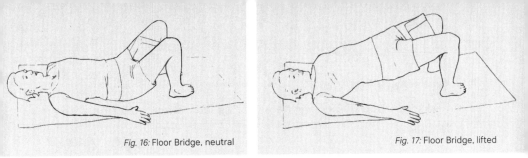

Fig. 16: Floor Bridge, neutral   *Fig. 17:* Floor Bridge, lifted

3. As you inhale, reverse the sequence, lowering your mid back, lower back, pelvis, and tailbone back to the floor. As much as possible, articulate your spine. Avoid moving in chunks. Imagine a string of pearls, and try to move and feel the pearl of each vertebra as your move.
4. Repeat this slowly five times.

Week Three

Add Cat Sitting on Ball.

CAT SITTING ON BALL

1. Sit on a ball with feet hip distance apart and place one hand on either thigh (see fig. 18).
2. When you exhale, curl your pelvis and drop your head forward, rounding your back (see fig. 19).
3. When you inhale, return to upright.
4. Repeat the cycle five times.

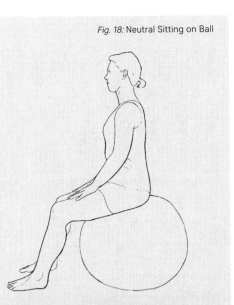

Fig. 18: Neutral Sitting on Ball

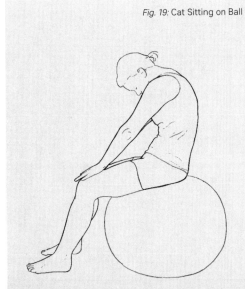

Fig. 19: Cat Sitting on Ball

Week Four

Add Interlaced Fingers (yoga asana called *badam gulyasana*) and Neck Roll.

INTERLACED FINGERS (BADAM GULYASANA) AND NECK ROLL

1. Interlace your fingers together, turn your palms away from you, and reach your arms over your head (see fig. 20).
2. Straighten your elbows and extend your arms, feeling your whole waist and rib cage lengthening.
3. Release your hands and slowly let your arms come down.
4. With your hands on your thighs, lean your head toward your right shoulder and lightly press your left hand into your thigh (see fig. 21).
5. Stay there and inhale.
6. When you exhale, roll your head to the other side.
7. Repeat the cycle five times.

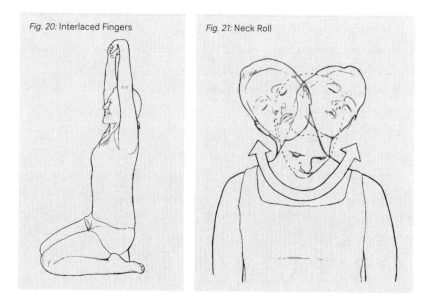

Fig. 20: Interlaced Fingers   *Fig. 21:* Neck Roll

Week Five

Add Reclining Foot in Strap (*supta padangusthasana* variation) and Reclining Butterfly (*supta buddhakonasana* variation).

RECLINING FOOT IN STRAP (SUPTA PADANGUSTHASANA VARIATION)

1. Lie down with your knees bent and feet flat on the floor. Place your feet together so your inner legs are touching.
2. Activate your lower belly with your exhale, and tip your pelvis so your whole lower back is pressed against the floor. Place a strap around the ball of your right foot, holding one end of the strap in either hand, and raise your right foot toward the ceiling (see fig. 22).
3. Keep your knees touching and roll your thighbones slightly inward, pulling the strap to feel a strong sensation in your calf. (This will probably not be a strong hamstring stretch; this is to feel connection from your leg to your abdomen and to clear stagnation in the lower legs, rather than a hamstring stretch.)
4. Hold for two minutes each side. Relax for at least a minute before moving on.

RECLINING BUTTERFLY (SUPTA BUDDHAKONASANA VARIATION)

1. For the next variation, maintain your lower back firmly pressing into the floor, and open your knees away from each other, bringing the soles of the feet together (see fig. 23). Don't let your knees flop open. If you do, your lower back will lift. Keep your knees as high as they need to be so you can maintain your lower back against the ground.
2. Hold for three to five minutes. It is normal for your legs to tremble. This is a good sign and means the little muscles are waking up.

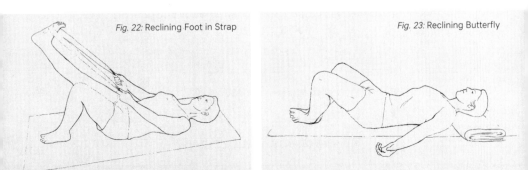

Fig. 22: Reclining Foot in Strap

Fig. 23: Reclining Butterfly

Week Six

Add Head Cradle, Eagle Arms (*garudasana* arms), and Reverse Prayer (*paschima namaskara*).

HEAD CRADLE

1. Sitting on the ball or in any sitting position, interlace your hands behind your head.
2. When you inhale, lift your chest and let your head rest back into your hands, arching your upper back. When you exhale, drop your chin to your chest, letting your elbows come toward each other. Make sure to keep your lower back stable and isolate the movement in your upper back (see fig. 24).
3. Repeat five times.

EAGLE ARMS (GARUDASANA ARMS)

1. Sitting on the ball, reach your arms forward at shoulder height.
2. Bend your elbows to ninety degrees. Place your right elbow into the crook of your left, and wind your forearms around each other until your palms touch (see fig. 25). If your palms don't touch, press the back of your hands together.
3. Squeeze your arms together, lift your elbows, and direct your attention and your breath between your shoulder blades.

REVERSE PRAYER (PASCHIMA NAMASKARA)

1. Hold opposite elbows behind your back (see fig. 26) or make a prayer position with your hands behind your back (see fig. 27). If you have tendinitis in your elbows or wrists or carpal tunnel, then take the first option, holding opposite elbows.
2. Broaden your chest and breathe into this posture. As you inhale, feel your collarbones spreading and broaden your chest.
3. Keep connecting to your lower belly on your exhale.

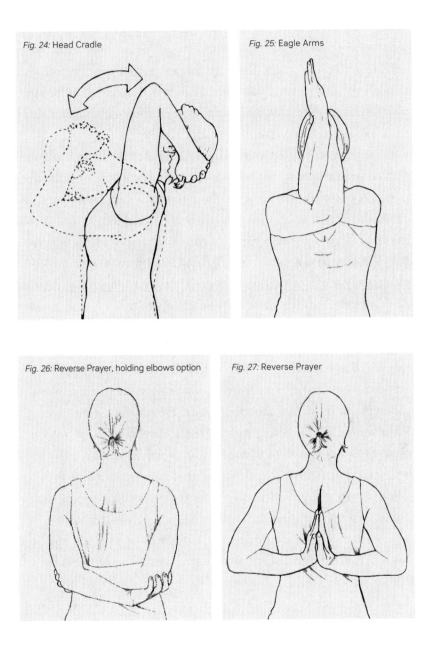

Fig. 24: Head Cradle

Fig. 25: Eagle Arms

Fig. 26: Reverse Prayer, holding elbows option

Fig. 27: Reverse Prayer

Carry Your Baby with Comfort

With greater pelvic support in place and experience in core engagement, new mothers will be able to lift, carry, and wear their babies with less strain on their lower backs. Inspired by indigenous and nomadic women around the world who carry their children throughout the day as they cook and work, women these days want to keep their babies close and have their hands free.

There are many benefits to baby wearing. For the baby, being carried close to the mother's body is an extension of the womb experience. Cocooned, the baby can hear mother's heartbeat, smell her chest and breast milk, and feel the familiar cadence of the mother's walk. This helps to organize a baby's nervous system. Because a baby's system and a mother's system are so interwoven at this time, we can say that the mother and baby are in a dynamic process of co-regulation. Studies show that babies actually cry less when they are worn. Baby wearing came into public awareness in the early 1980s, when Dr. Harvey Karp studied a South African tribe whose babies did not experience colic. He found that the main reason those babies rarely cried was because they were always in close physical contact with other humans who carried them.

For moms, it's liberating to have the ability to shop for groceries, cook, do laundry, and go to the bathroom, while keeping baby close and safe. Babies love this closeness that often puts them to sleep. There are so many carriers on the market, some that support ergonomic function for mom and baby alike, and others that do not. It is important to find at least one style that works best for you and your baby. Because the core is not as strong as usual after having a baby, it can be a bit of double whammy to then carry weight without good underlying support. Taking some time to try out various styles, even before the birth but certainly once the baby is born, can save you money, and emotional and physical stress. Some birthing-related stores will rent carriers for a week at a time so you can experiment with a particular style before purchasing. Note that carriers that keep your baby's limbs tucked in and spine in its natural concave curve are more appropriate for a newborn, versus ones that encourage the baby's limbs, especially legs, to dangle and chest to push forward. You'll want your newborn's carrier to help mimic the warm embrace of your arms during these early days in life.

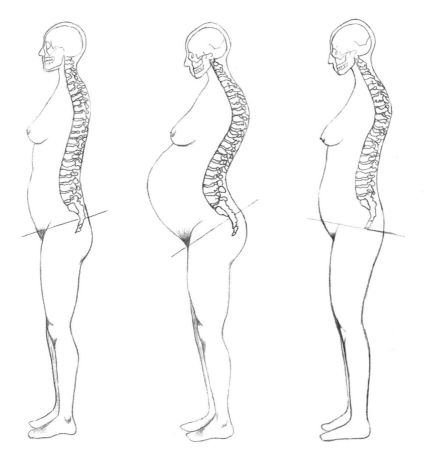

Fig. 28: Postural profiles: before pregnancy, during pregnancy, and postpartum

Whenever you use the baby carrier, take care to distort your posture as little as possible. For instance, if you are wearing your baby backpack style, be careful not to jut your head forward. If you are wearing your baby in a sling on one side, notice if you are throwing that hip out as well. If you are wearing your baby in the front, don't tuck your pelvis and push your hips forward. If you are able to pay attention to your plumb line and keep your pelvic floor engaged to support you, baby-wearing can turn into an amazing toning and strengthening exercise. If the weight is too much, and you are compensating to be able to manage carrying your baby, you may end up with pain from the repetitive stress of your postural shifts, taking you out of alignment.

When you are carrying your baby, the closer he or she is to your body, the better. With the baby's body tight to your center of gravity, it will seem like you are carrying a lighter load. If you plan to wear your baby a lot, it's smart to have a few options in carriers, so you can vary the demands on your body. Changing the ways you tie the carrier you have or changing the carrier itself will give your body a chance to adapt to different weight-distribution patterns. Some variety will help to alleviate accumulated tension and fatigue that happens if the same area is being taxed over and over and will allow you to maintain healthy posture.

Taking into account the benefits that baby wearing may have for your baby and you, it is still okay to be honest about the toll that baby wearing can take on your body. If you are experiencing a lot of lower back, pelvic, or neck pain, you may want to consider how you are carrying your baby. If you have made the necessary adjustments with the carrier and are sure that you are wearing it correctly, have tried a couple of types, and are still experiencing discomfort, or if you had a birth injury or preexisting injury, then you may need to take a break and do some rehabilitative movement first.

I carried my daughter all over Rio de Janeiro until she was three years old in an Ergo backpack carrier. I lived in a neighborhood with cobblestone streets. On a stroller ride, her head bounced around so much, I worried about giving her a minor head injury. Padding the side of her head did not stop her from being jolted around on a simple walk. There were so many rocks, bumps, and divots in the sidewalks that on a short walk, when I hadn't adequately strapped her in, she actually went catapulting into the street. Walking down subway steps and getting in and out of taxis with a stroller were also deterrents.

However, mostly I just couldn't give myself a break. Even though I grabbed my back, braced my hands on my thighs to get up and down off the ground, and groaned for the first two years of her life, my idea of being a good mother was wearing her. I was in the most physical pain I had ever experienced in my life, but I didn't stop to question if wearing her was costing me more than she was gaining. I just continued imagining that I would find a way to fix myself later. I know now that my recovery would have been a lot different had I had access to postpartum rehabilitation exercises in those first couple of years. But I didn't have the knowledge that I have now, and I learned through experience that I did not have to resign myself to being in pain or sacrifice my posture to be a good mother.

I saw pictures of women from all over the world carrying their children, and I didn't want to transport my baby and toddler from box to box, car seat to stroller to crib. I wanted her to feel the rhythm of natural movement and benefit from the closeness. Yet I didn't take into account two very important factors. First, most of the women in the pictures I saw lived in a tribal context. Therefore, the birth mother didn't carry the baby all the time. Babies are passed between other children, sisters and cousins, aunts and grandmothers throughout the day. Second, the lifestyles of women in these tribes lent themselves to having a stronger base of core support. These women squatted while getting water, planting seeds, gathering crops, cooking. Many of them don't wear underwear, which requires them to have a different and often more active relationship to their pelvic floor. Most of them have unmedicated vaginal births and, therefore, don't run the same risks of tearing and complicated recoveries that we do. Yes, I was an accomplished yoga teacher and a person who moved a lot, especially without a car living in a big city, but I still did not live my life in a tribal context, with my days in movement and in relationship to the earth.

I find that baby wearing is one of the places where new moms get into a martyr pattern. Even if they are feeling terrible in their bodies, they feel they must bear with it, stick through it, and sacrifice themselves for the good of the baby. This is just one area in mothering where we have the opportunity to look at our own conditioning and recognize what underlies the decisions we are making. It is also another chance to walk the middle path.

BODYWORK AFTER BIRTH

Did you know as women we can never be too kind to ourselves?
—MAYA TIWARI

There is no such thing as being too pampered or being treated too well (that goes for your newborn too). In our utilitarian culture, that which is not essential is considered a luxury. But what if I told you that postpartum touch actually is a necessity? Daily touch can often be the difference between surviving and thriving, the difference between depression and connectedness.

After giving birth, you may feel like you ran a marathon, or some women say they feel like they were run over by a truck. I hope you feel better than both of those examples; however, whatever your experience was and is, you have been through a *major* bodily event. Your body went through something that had its own particular nuances and qualities based on the environment you were in, the company you held, and the body you brought with you into the birth. The length of your labor, how close to your due date you were, and how the birth matched your expectations can all contribute to how you are feeling in your body.

Bodywork can help to keep you grounded at a time when you can feel very expansive but also a little unstable. For the first couple of weeks, the best form of bodywork is something nourishing and settling that takes into account your energy body as well as your physical body. Your organs and muscles are still returning to their regular sizes and spaces; your hormones are still recalibrating (and will continue to).

Helpful Bodywork during the Fourth Trimester

As mentioned earlier, standard postpartum health care for women is a short visit to the doctor or midwife at the six-week mark. Beyond that, I recommend that every woman invest in an appointment with a pelvic-floor physical therapist or STREAM practitioner at this stage as well, someone whom she hopefully saw before or during pregnancy. While it may seem like a big investment of time and money, this specialized care will offer accurate information and, just as important, peace of mind. Women need to know more than if their stitches have dissolved or if their uterus is in the right place. Because many doctors don't have many solutions to offer other than surgery, they often minimize diagnoses or leave women feeling helpless or, worse, crazy. I have worked with dozens of women who felt like things "weren't right down there," only to be told that everything was "fine."

Another common response that women receive from care providers is to wait, see if things go back to normal, and come back in a year. If things are not normal in a year, they will assess for surgery. A wait-and-see approach to pelvic health is negligent and ultimately damaging. If a woman is experiencing painful sex, pain at the tearing or incision site, heaviness or bulging, or simply seeing or feeling things at their vaginal entrance that were never there before, there are many holistic approaches to take before considering a surgical intervention, which may not even be effective for the aforementioned problems.

Helpful bodywork includes, but is not limited to:

Ayurvedic oil massage (abhyanga);

Swedish massage;

hot-stone massage;

acupuncture;

craniosacral therapy;

Feldenkrais technique;

holistic pelvic core (see www.wildfeminine.com);

Mayan abdominal massage;

osteopathy; and

STREAM pelvic health care (see www.scartissueremediation.com)

Bodywork therapies to avoid during the fourth trimester include:

deep-tissue massage;

Rolfing/Structural Integration; and

Thai massage.

While you may feel structurally out of alignment, this is not the time to go for aggressive chiropractic adjustments or deep-tissue massage, even if that is generally your bodywork of choice. During the immediate postpartum time, if you feel the need for structural adjustments, the best options are osteopathy, craniosacral work, or network chiropractic—all methods that take into account the subtle body as well as bony movement.

Physical Therapists

A physical therapist will be able to give you clear feedback. She or he has machines that measure strength and activation of your pelvic-floor muscles. A physical therapist will also be able to assess where you are in your healing process. Every woman's healing process is different. Not every woman is "loose" in her vaginal and pelvic-floor muscles after giving birth. I have worked with women who were actually very tense, and their muscles had spasmed, becoming tighter after labor. Your pelvic floor needs attention even if you have had a cesarean delivery. A physical therapist will be able to offer you the right exercises for your body and give you a specific protocol concerning how to move forward toward repair and wholeness.

A holistic pelvic care practitioner will include an energetic component to treatment.

Massage

During the fourth trimester, I also strongly recommend either Ayurvedic abhyanga or Swedish massage. Both of these styles use oils and give you a sense of satisfying contact. Your body is changing rapidly, and it is very useful to stay in contact with how you feel inside your body during these changes. Since your body size and shape have changed rapidly, it is satisfying and helpful to feel your contours and the outline of your body, and massage helps with circulation, lymphatic drainage, and flushing out toxins. Oil massage can also help to settle your nervous system, helping you sleep better.

Right now, you want to be lavished and lathered with satisfying contact that leaves you feeling replenished. This time for bodywork is just for you and goes a long way to building your resources during this time of unpredictable sleep and changing demands from your baby.

Postpartum Doulas

Postpartum doulas are trained to know and serve the physiological and emotional needs of new mothers. Many women dismiss postpartum doula services as a luxury, not understanding that a postpartum doula is much more than a glorified housekeeper or night nurse. A great postpartum doula can attend to all of the universal postpartum needs: preparing fresh, nourishing food, appropriate bodywork, leading you in breath exercises, wrapping your belly, reminding you to rest, making your house beautiful, and listening to you. Investing in your care at this time sets you up for a peaceful recovery where you feel nurtured and strong, so that you can nurture your baby. Many women say that their partner is taking a week or two off work, and that should be enough. A postpartum doula also lightens the load on partners, so that both mother and partner can focus on nurturing the baby and experiencing the precious time together. There will be plenty of time when you will be on your own, taking care of everything yourself. Training for postpartum doulas is widely varied. When hiring a postpartum doula, ask them what their background and focus are to make sure they are trained in the areas of care you are most interested in receiving.

Avoid Having Too Many "Experts"

Many of the moms who contact me are receiving all kinds of treatments, some with commitments almost every day. Some days it's the pediatrician, other days acupuncture, other days the lactation consultant, yet still others massage. While it is wonderful to be able to receive care, so much varied input and advice can be confusing and disorganizing. New moms often feel anxious, and rather than rest at home and receive consistent treatments from a single trusted practitioner, they are scrambling around, trying to find answers to problems that may not even be there if they were moving less—and if there were less advice from so many different people. Just as spiritual texts say that a great teacher points you to the answers inside yourself, a great postpartum care provider helps a new mother listen to her own inner guidance.

A Special Note on C-Section Recovery

A cesarean section is major abdominal surgery. With any other major surgery, a doctor would prescribe rehabilitation. Imagine getting knee surgery, then being sent home with some painkillers and that's it for six weeks—no rehab or other care instructions. For some reason, no rehabilitation is considered standard for a C-section, though it is a major surgery. You will be taking medicine to manage the pain, and therefore should *underestimate* your ability to do activities. The pain medication masks the feelings of pain to your brain, not letting you experience what your body is actually going through to repair itself. So wait until you are finished with your pain medications to start any of the movement plan. You will be advised to walk some, to maintain the circulation in your legs, but restrict this to walking around your house.

Always roll to your side when getting out of bed, and use your hands, rather than your abdominal muscles, to press up to sitting position. Avoid sitting up with your head first or jerking yourself up with momentum. Ask for help when getting up and sitting or lying down. Many women assume that because they did not have a vaginal delivery, their pelvic floor was not affected. This is not true. Your pelvic floor was still a support for your organs and the baby the entire time he or she was in your belly. Even if you had a scheduled cesarean, you still need to begin your post-birth healing with the breath for length and core-restoration exercises.

The belly wrap is especially important in C-section deliveries to help provide support to all the layers that were cut through, and especially to help the connective tissue weave back together. Wear it as soon as you get home from the hospital. It will also help you carry your baby with less discomfort and additional strain. Don't lift anything heavy for the first six weeks or so.

After your scar is healed, *uddiyana bandha kriya*—as taught in chapter 11—is an important practice to care for your scar, together with castor oil packs and massage.

SUMMARY

- Gentle restorative movement is the place to start in the fourth trimester.
- Beginning exercise too soon can cause setbacks in the healing process.
- Bodywork is a necessary part of the healing process for new moms.

Reflections

- Are you receiving enough touch? If not, whom can you ask for it—a trusted friend, your partner, a professional bodyworker?
- What support do you need to be able to follow this week-by-week movement plan? When and where will you do it each day?
- Is there anything that feels like it may not be healing just right and needs special attention? Take out your sanctuary plan and call the person you need.

Practices

- Follow the week-by-week movement plan.
- Make a six-week postpartum physical-therapy appointment in addition to your checkup with your ob-gyn.
- Wrap your belly and hips.

8

understanding
medical realities

The midwives are between my legs. My baby is on my chest, her dad beside me. It's been some time since I delivered the placenta. But since they are still down there, I start to realize something is wrong.

"Did I tear?"

"Yes, a little bit, but we'll stitch you up."

After twenty-six hours of unmedicated labor, I get a shot of local anesthetic in my perineum. Yet I still feel the tugging of the stitches, together with the stinging of my nipples from my baby trying to nurse and the sharp uterine contractions as she suckles. It's a lot of sensation to track at once.

I'm not experiencing the elation and tears I expected I would. I'm relieved and starting to feel worried. It's taking them a long time to stitch me up, which tells me it's pretty bad. When I ask how many stitches, they say that they didn't count. When I ask exactly where, they say, "Everything's going to be okay."

I'm not satisfied with this answer. I have mapped every centimeter of my own body through years of dance, yoga, bodywork, and sitting meditation practice. I want to know exactly what is happening. I can't feel much, so I want them to help me fill in the gaps, but there is so much going on. My parents arrive. "What's the baby's name?" they ask.

I feel totally unprepared to answer that question. All I can think is, *What happened to my body?*

Many women tell me that they had absolutely no idea that what they experienced during birth or are experiencing postpartum was even possible. As a birth educator, one of the biggest questions I face is how much to tell pregnant women about what can potentially happen during and after birth. I don't want to scare anyone. At the same time, I do want to save women the despair and disillusionment of experiencing symptoms that they have never heard of and had no idea were possible. In most cases, it is not just the pain of the actual dysfunction or injury that troubles women—it is the feelings of confusion and isolation.

While nothing can take away the pain of an injury, the suffering can be minimized when a woman has sufficient information and some context for what happened to her. In this chapter, we'll go over some medical realities that are common after childbirth. While they are *common*, they are not *normal*. The bad news is that there are some possible physical outcomes of childbirth that require special attention and rehabilitation, and may take time to heal. The good news is that while many practitioners, from doctors to physical therapists, may say that it is just something to manage or live with, or to take a "wait and see" approach, there is a lot of healing that you can do to return to healthy function and feel whole again that does not include surgery. While you may feel broken, it is not permanent. Some bodies take longer than others to repair, but your birth outcome is not a life sentence, and you are not alone. It may take more time than feels fair or convenient, but healing is possible.

ANTICIPATE THE SIX-WEEK CHECKUP

After giving birth, most women will see their doctor or midwife once or twice in the following days. Then, several weeks will pass with no professional support at all. During this time, as women are getting to know their babies, they are also experiencing the profound aftereffects of their birth experience. The medical realities of this period can come as a surprise to many women. To make matters worse, women generally don't talk to each other about these realities.

Typically, the six-week postpartum doctor's visit will only clear women for returning to exercise or having sex. What they leave out is most everything else. Hemorrhoids, structural pain, incontinence, pain at stitching, prolapse, and emotional distress are a few of the symptoms included in the range of "normal." Often women who are given the go-ahead to exercise and make love don't feel remotely ready for either. Many women are offered the birth control pill or antidepressants at their postpartum checkups; some of my clients have been offered both at the same time. While some women may want or need one or both of these medications, using hormonal treatment for every kind of symptom, including physical injuries, is a mistake. This practice reflects the brokenness of the medical model that isn't equipped to look at the whole picture, but instead divides our experience into pieces and parts. Most obstetricians are not trained to evaluate the structural or biomechanical health and integrity of the pelvic floor—but physical therapists are. Unfortunately right now, referrals to physical therapists are the exception rather than the rule, so each woman needs to advocate for herself to receive this important piece of health care.

I have heard from many women that their postpartum checkups took less than ten minutes. To remedy possible confusion and get a thorough evaluation, I recommend that women go to a postpartum physical-therapy, holistic pelvic care, or STREAM session in addition to their six-week checkup with a doctor or midwife. Don't be afraid to ask your doctor for a referral even if everything seems okay. That way, you can ask all the questions you may have and get a clear picture of how the healing process is going from someone whose expertise is pelvic health. It is the therapist's job to take you through a thorough assessment, answer your questions, and ask you any questions that may have been overlooked.

Unfortunately, with the way our health-care system is set up, many birth doctors don't have much follow-up with their patients. When they make interventions during labor and birth, whether it's anesthetic, forceps, or vacuum delivery, episiotomies or doing repairs, they don't have long-term follow-up with women to see how their lives have been affected. I attended a birth as a doula where the doctor pulled the baby out with forceps. In order to use forceps, there is almost always an episiotomy, or vaginal incision, to make more room for the instruments. In this particular birth, the incision extended into a tear through the whole pelvic floor. The doctor looked over at me, shrugged, and matter-of-factly said, "The rectal sphincter popped, but we just sew it back up." I knew that this doctor would probably not see this woman again, so he most likely would not know what the future ramifications of this intervention would be for her.

Statistically, 75 percent of women will experience some kind of pelvic-floor dysfunction after a childbirth that includes a mechanical intervention, such as forceps or vacuum extraction. I know from working with women in my office and from personal experience that it can take years to recover from the aftereffects of these kinds of injuries. The problem is that they are not categorized as injuries. If they were, women would be referred to physical therapy routinely after birth.

In many cases, the six-week checkup is supposed to be the beginning of a recovery phase after birth, but more often, it signals the end of midwifery or doctor care. I see women week in and week out in my practice suffering from pelvic-floor dysfunction who feel abandoned by their birth practitioners. They are too embarrassed to ask their primary-care physicians about fecal incontinence or painful sex, and often their problems remain unaddressed. If they do share that something doesn't feel right, often the doctor or midwife simply says everything is fine and will get better over time. To arm and empower you, some of these issues are outlined and defined in what follows, so you will have a better idea of what to look out for and talk about with your health-care professionals.

THE FOUR DOMAINS OF PELVIC HEALTH

We arrive at the birth altar with the same body that has carried us to this point. Every moment we have lived—though our minds may have forgotten, may not have been present, or may have been anesthetized—our bodies were there. Your body never left you and is a trustworthy living record of all you have experienced. Therefore, the body has all of the organic intelligence and the keys to your healing. After a lifetime of conditioning that tells us we can think our way into answers and understanding, our first step after giving birth is to come back into deep contact with our body.

The next step is to befriend our bodies and learn to listen to their signals. Listening to the language of our bodies is an ongoing process, but it brings us into direct relationship with the parts of ourselves that know what we need in order to heal. Rather than looking outside for answers, we become our own inner authority, our own inner doctor. We begin to understand what we actually need, rather than what we think we need. There is no greater tool for mothering than an authentic connection to our own sensations, emotions, and the truths communicated through them.

Although we may want to know why things happen, we may never know the exact reason for why we are injured, why we tore, why our abdominal muscles separated, or why everything seemed totally fine and now is not. There is rarely one discrete cause for one discrete symptom; there are constellations of moments that converge to create particular outcomes. Unraveling those constellations to connect the dots of one's story is part of our evolution as humans, women, and mothers.

When it comes to pelvic health, there are four domains that hold the key to our healing. Most medical and health-care professionals are trained to look at just one or two of these areas. But when we take all four into account, we have a powerful combination to accurately address pelvic-floor symptoms in a meaningful and lasting way.

You may feel great in three of the areas, but the one you haven't considered could be the root cause of whatever your symptom is. These four basic elements of health are biomechanics, biochemistry, emotions, and scar tissue. I first learned about the model of the four domains (see fig. 29) from my mentor, Ellen Heed, PhD. She developed this model to serve the needs of women who had painful sex from pelvic-floor scar tissue after giving birth. The key to your health, healing, and self-understanding lies in your understanding of these four domains.

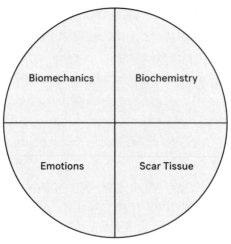

Fig 29: The Four Domains of Pelvic Health

Biomechanics

You can think of biomechanics as posture and flexibility. How you stand affects the position of your pelvic floor. Pregnancy and childbirth often exaggerate the postural tendencies that you already had. If you already had a swayback, you may notice that your lower back curve gets even more pronounced. If you rounded your upper back and pushed your thighs and hips forward, you may find yourself doing this even more. We live in the field of gravity. Posture determines whether the impact of gravity is working for us creating a sense of life and buoyancy, or against us creating a sense of heaviness and descent. Your genetics play a part in your flexibility; the way you move and hold yourself is in part a result of the density or stretchiness of your connective tissue. When your spine has its natural lumbar curve, your pelvic organs have a little shelf on your pubic bones. If you have a pronounced curve in your low back, your uterus may get pushed onto your bladder, in turn pushing your bladder too far toward your vaginal canal. If you are tucking your pelvis and flattening your buttocks, the bladder and uterus lose their shelf of support and this can contribute to pelvic-floor dysfunction like prolapse and incontinence.

Biochemistry

Biochemistry describes the internal environment of your body. It's mostly influenced by your diet and nutrition, but it is also influenced by exposure to pollutants, what you take into your body through food, and how that food is absorbed. Are your tissues hydrated? How is your blood moving? What medicines have you taken in the past or present? Have you had prior surgeries and been under anesthesia? What kind of anesthetic did you use during birth? Is there inflammation in your system? Inflammation causes biochemical changes in tissues that irritate nerves and cause pain.

As mentioned in chapter 6, postpartum women need healthy saturated fats, adequate hydration, and whole foods to rebuild what was lost in pregnancy and childbirth. Collagen- and mineral-rich foods are two elements common to indigenous diets that are specific to postpartum women. For all women, but especially women with less connective tissue density, saturated fats from grass-fed cream and butter and other animal protein are imperative to giving the body the basic building blocks to strengthen organ tissue and ligaments, and return them to a robust and stable structure.

In proper Darwinian fashion, the body will take whatever it needs from the mother to make the highest-quality breast milk possible for the baby. In order to heal well after childbirth, it is crucial that women have sufficient nutrient density to nourish both themselves and their babies, especially if added healing is needed. Maintaining even blood-sugar levels by eating three balanced meals with two snacks will also help ensure that a woman is getting the building blocks she needs to recover.

Biochemistry also includes hormones. As described in chapter 5, after delivering the placenta there is a steep drop in progesterone and estrogen as the body shifts toward healing and milk production. While pregnant, your placenta was making these hormones; after delivery, your ovaries have to kick back into gear. Sometimes thyroid, adrenal, or pituitary imbalances appear after giving birth. If you have a history of hormonal imbalance, which could manifest as painful periods, fertility challenges, or depression, or have been on the pill to regulate symptoms, you want to take care to have blood work done so that you can confirm that your body has returned to making the hormones that you need. Likewise, if you have a history of depression or anxiety, and feel these states activated, make sure to ask for an evaluation from your doctor so that you can feel safe, secure, and stable. You may need to seek out a naturopathic doctor or a specialist in functional medicine to get the tests you need.

Emotions

Emotion plays a role in healing most tangibly when women have had either preexisting trauma or birth trauma itself. Whatever is happening at the time an injury is sustained is an important factor for healing that injury. The domain of emotion also includes our ability to self-regulate, to care for, and to soothe ourselves when experiencing the unknown or during times of difficulty.

It's impossible to talk about post-birth medical realities without taking into consideration the very specific emotional, spiritual, and psychological nature of pelvic-floor dysfunction. Women use words like *broken*, *damaged*, and even *eviscerated* to describe how they feel. Because these injuries are typically invisible and occur in territory that is rarely explored, they remain untreated, but not unfelt.

Some of us may have shame that prevents us from exploring or seeking care for these injuries. Many women don't want to explain to their partners how they are feeling because they don't want their partners to see them as damaged or unlovable. They don't want their partners to avoid sex with them and view them as damaged. One client shared, "I can't think of anything less appealing than him knowing that my bladder is falling out of my vagina. Why would I want him to know that? He can't feel it while I am on my back. I prefer to leave it that way." Feeling damaged in the pelvic floor can make some women consciously or unconsciously want to avoid sex, creating confusion when there is no language to describe their injury's location or sensation, or a total fear of communicating their physical reality to a partner.

Many women have never met anyone who has openly discussed the symptoms they are feeling. Walking around in daily life with organs that feel like they are falling out, or with bumpy and rough skin where it was once smooth, or with a fear of wetting our pants or pooping in them creates a nonstop internal commentary, with the symptom always present in the background. It can make women avoid many behaviors and situations they would normally participate in, from running to sitting with open legs to having sex.

Emotions play a key role in memory formation. Disentangling the emotion from the physical injury is often a key piece of healing, and is why working only with the biomechanics isn't always effective.

Scar Tissue

To understand scar tissue, we first need to understand connective tissue, or fascia.

Fascia is the wrapping of the body. If you think of an orange and peeling back the skin, underneath it, the whole orange remains intact because of the pith, the white part. Divide the orange in half and it will remain intact because of the deeper layer of pith. Then, when you divide it into fourths and eventually individual pieces, each will be wrapped, all the way down to each piece of pulp. The body is similar; if you were to remove our skin, we are wrapped in a sheath of connective tissue. Then each muscle group, each muscle, and finally each muscle fiber is also wrapped in layers of this gauzelike tissue. What we want is for these layers to be able slide over each other. When we experience muscle knots, often it is wadded-up connective tissue that is not sliding easily. When it lets go and softens, what is inside the wrapping can reorganize. The body-wide web of fascia is connected to everything else in the body, which explains why, when touched in one area, we can feel a connection to another area in our body.

This tissue is made up of several kinds of fiber, including collagen and elastin fibers. Elastin fibers make fascia pliable and elastic, as the name suggests. Collagen fibers make the tissue resilient, strong, and dense. We all have a different ratio of elastin and collagen fibers in our connective tissue, due mostly to genetics. More elastic tissue will stretch farther without tearing but will have a harder time coming back together when torn. Collagenous tissue won't have as much give and may tear more easily, but it will lay down collagen fibers to repair itself faster.

Scar tissue isn't on the radar of most health-care providers, yet it is a key player in many women's pelvic-health issues. Over 80 percent of women come through childbirth with some kind of scar tissue in their pelvis. Scar tissue looks and feels like a brittle chaotic spider web, with crisscrossed fibers and little pebbles or rocks inside it. It can also feel like stringy rope or be very dense and thick, like rubbery calamari. Imagine layers of plastic wrap smashed together, almost impossible to peel apart without tearing. Tissue that was once fluid, glistening, and pulsing in rhythm with breath and blood circulation becomes dehydrated, immobile, and unable to pulse at the same rhythm as the rest of the organism. Healthy fascia has a certain ratio of collagen fibers to elastin fibers, but scar tissue has a disproportionate amount of collagen fibers to bind where it was cut, torn, or damaged.

Scar tissue can be formed from birth tears, stitched repairs, C-sections, episiotomies, forceps or vacuum deliveries, babies being stuck in certain positions for long periods of time in the pelvis, the force of the pushing phase, or expulsion itself putting specific pressure on tissues in the pelvis. Women often have preexisting pelvic scar tissue from gynecological procedures, surgeries, miscarriages, abortions, endometriosis, or sexual abuse.

Scars are physical artifacts of trauma. Often emotions come up when scar tissue is touched for the first time. Gentle, persistent touch will allow the scar to begin to let go. It is normal for there to be sensitivity and numbness. Often, there is tingling and vibration as sensation begins to return to the area of the scar. It is important to touch the scar non-aggressively and allow the tissue the time it needs to soften. Understand that scars that are not tended to can potentially grow, forming more adhesions, which can affect circulation, organ placement, and even posture.

Even though there are a lot of ways that we may accumulate scar tissue, we can also dissolve it. Both movement and heat can contribute to the dissolution of the scar tissue. The body then flushes with blood, lymph, and hydration and is able to carry away the collagen fibers that are no longer needed, replacing them with healthy, new structures and enabling reorganization to occur. That means that scars can become elastic and pliable and even completely disintegrate.

Castor oils packs are the most effective way to begin the process of reorganizing scar tissue. Start by saturating organic cotton flannel strips with castor oil and placing them over the affected area—the abdomen or perineum. Place a hot-water bottle over the soaked strips and let it sit for about twenty minutes. Then, massage the castor oil into the scar tissue for a few minutes, until it is absorbed. Do this every day, or at least most days, for a minimum of three weeks.

If the scar tissue is internal, you can soak an organic cotton tampon in organic castor oil and place it inside your vagina for twenty minutes. After you remove the tampon, use your fingers or a wand or dildo to work on the scar tissue internally. Do this every other day, rather than every day. Women can be sensitive to castor oil inside their vagina, and using castor oil every other day helps avoid sensitization for most women. It is also helpful to work with a professional who may be able to get angles that are hard for you to reach yourself, to assess the trail of the scar, and to provide instruction, so your full experience can be guided.

SOME OF THE MEDICAL REALITIES

After giving birth, I experienced the following symptoms and medical realities: incontinence, diastasis, tearing, and prolapse. My own healing process required years of dedicated exploration and trial and error, as well as major life changes. I had no idea what factors were contributing to my recovery. I felt profoundly broken. For months I could not sit or nurse my baby from an upright position. I could not walk well so I had to minimize trips outside. I was isolated, living far away from my language, my country, and all that was familiar. The pain from the scar, which did not heal correctly, contributed to a downward spiral of problems. I was not producing enough breast milk from all the stress, and was fighting against supplementing with milk from other sources. My lower back and sacroiliac joints hurt all the time. My hip joints felt loose, like they might just keep meandering farther and farther away from each other, until they walked off in separate directions. My organs felt like they were about to fall onto the ground. I went from someone who was having sex almost every day while I was pregnant to someone who couldn't conceive of having sex at all. When I decided to try despite my body's aversion to engage sexually, it was incredibly painful and reinforced my feelings of being damaged and that something was seriously wrong. Worse yet, everyone I asked for help—my midwives and lactation consultants—acted like nothing was that bad, that it was all "normal." Deep down I knew, as many women do, that everything was definitely not normal—common, perhaps, but not normal. Yet I still had no idea what to do about it.

First, I had to understand exactly what was going on, and it took years to parse out the various factors that were contributing to my pain and dysfunction. Below is a glossary with detailed definitions of each issue. While I hope that you experience none of the symptoms that I did, I want you to have the information so that, if you do encounter one of them, you are able to recognize it and get the help you need.

Incontinence

Incontinence is the medical term describing involuntary leakage of urine or feces. Urinary incontinence is when urine escapes the bladder. Peeing, even if just a little bit, when jumping or coughing or sneezing is called *stress incontinence.* Not being able to hold it when your bladder is full or just feeling like you have to urinate all the time is called *urge incontinence.* Urinary incontinence is common, but it is not normal. For many women, it glides under their radar. When I ask women who come to see me for structural bodywork how their pelvic floors are doing, most give me a bit of a confused look and say fine. A bit later, they might say, "Well, actually, I have to really concentrate, squeeze my legs together, and hope for the best every time I cough." But since no one has ever asked them the question and their symptoms are not that bad, they just accept it as normal. Many women would never think of jumping rope or getting on a trampoline after having a child, but they have adjusted their lifestyles without noticing it. It's easy to understand why. Raising children, working, managing relationships, trying to get in some exercise—they all trump taking real stock of unseen symptoms until they are so blatant that they are impossible to ignore. Simply put, we get used to living with the little inconveniences.

For the first few days after giving birth, it's normal to have a little bit of leakage. But if incontinence continues beyond those first few days, it doesn't typically get better on its own. Most people presume that if they have incontinence it is because their pelvic floor is too weak. They are told to do Kegels but not taught how to do them properly. In fact, about half the time, incontinence is caused by pelvic-floor muscles that are too tight, in which case, even a properly executed Kegel will not help. Scar tissue can also be a contributor to incontinence, as it can pull on the bladder or urethra, and other connected structures.

Continued incontinence requires the help of a physical therapist or sexological bodyworker who can help with hands-on work, breathing, and movement exercises.

Diastasis

A *diastasis* is a separation of the muscles of the outermost abdominal wall, the rectus abdominis (see fig. 30). The rectus abdominis is the six-pack muscle group that begins at the mid-ribs and attaches at the pubic bones—most people just call them "abs." They are divided in half down the middle by connective tissue called the *linea alba*. During pregnancy, with the weight of the baby putting pressure on the abdomen and stretching the abdominal wall, these muscles can separate and spread apart. After giving birth, the muscles can stay separated. The separation can occur anywhere between the sternum and the pubic bone. It is measured in fingertips' width distance that can fit into the separation, usually at three points along the linea alba—two above the navel and one below. It's most common that the biggest separation occurs by the belly button. It's normal to have one or two fingers' distance just after giving birth. Less important than the size of the diastasis is the density of connective tissue of the individual woman. It is possible to have a diastasis and still have full function and integrity in the linea alba.

Ideally, your doula or postpartum-care provider would manually check you for diastasis ten days to two weeks postpartum, so you

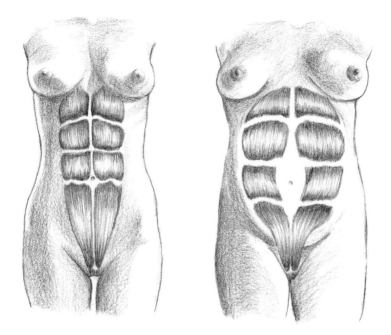

Fig. 30: Diastasis

would know to diligently wrap your belly and start the breath for length exercises. It is difficult to manually check for yourself; however, if you are lying down and lift your head, and your belly makes a cone shape or you see something bulging at the midline, then you probably have a diastasis. In that case, make sure to ask your practitioner or even a friend to check you.

Diastasis is most common in women with a very strong abdominal wall, such as rock climbers and triathletes. It is also common in yoga practitioners who backbend frequently while pregnant.

How to check for a diastasis:

1. Lie down with your knees bent and feet flat.
2. Have a friend kneel to your right. Have them place the four fingers of their right hand horizontally on the midline of your abdominals just below your ribs. They need to press down gently to feel where the linea alba is and how big the gap is in a resting position.

3. Next, lift your head up.
4. What happens to their fingers? Does the gap close, does it stay the same, or does it widen?
5. Repeat this process in three places—just below the ribs, just above the navel, and between the navel and the pubic bone.

A one-finger gap after a baby is okay. Any more than that will require targeted breathing exercises and, potentially, splinting. Knowing the three numbers will help you track your progress. You can check every week to see if the gap is closing.

There are specific movements for diastasis recovery, the most important of which is the diligent recruitment and entrainment of your transverse abdominis, your corset muscles, together with pelvic-floor activation. You want to lift your pelvic floor as the belly moves toward your spine, without tucking your pelvis. This movement is explained in the breath for length in chapter 4. The most comprehensive method for diastasis recovery is the Tuppler method, which combines targeted movement exercises together with abdominal splinting, and can be started whenever you discover you have one.

An intact abdominal wall protects soft organs. When the abdominal wall splits, there is potential for hernia. A diastasis can contribute to lower back pain, as well as an overall feeling of physical and emotional instability and vulnerability.

Tearing

As your baby comes through the birth canal, there is a tremendous amount of stretching that needs to happen. Sometimes the tissues don't have enough time to stretch sufficiently, or they are tight to begin with, and the skin or muscles tear. Tearing is measured in degrees. A first-degree tear is when the skin of the vagina, labia, or perineum tears. Often first-degree tears don't require stitches, but it's helpful to keep your legs together for ten days to two weeks, so the tissues continue to come together and don't re-tear. A second-degree tear goes through the skin and the underlying pelvic-floor and vaginal muscles. A third-degree tear goes through the skin and the muscles, all the way to the front of the anal sphincter. A fourth-degree tear goes all the way through all those layers as well as through the back of the anal sphincter, damaging rectal nerves. Second-, third-, and fourth-degree tears all require skillful layer-by-layer stitching to reconstruct and reconnect the tissues.

The stitching is done when the tissues are highly engorged. So when the swelling goes down, it is common that the texture of the tissue has changed or that things are not as symmetrical as they were before. It can be very disconcerting to feel that things are not at all back to normal, functionally or visually. The perineum can be bumpy rather than smooth. The introitus, or vaginal opening, can be asymmetrical, rather than round and even. Many women aren't sure how they looked or felt before, but they know that things are different after birth. For this reason, I recommend that all women take photos of their vulvas. I have even heard of a woman who took a picture of her vulva to the birth, so if she needed a repair, her midwife or doctor would know how she looked originally and help to return her as close as possible to how she was.

Tearing can be confusing because symptoms don't always correlate with the degree of tear. For instance, a second-degree tear can lead to more complications than a fourth-degree tear. This has to do with your particular connective-tissue density, how well you are able to rest during healing, how well the repair was done, and your past sexual and health history. I have worked with women who experienced fourth-degree tears but had such great repairs that, together with ample rest and recovery, they experienced no pelvic-floor dysfunction. I have also worked with women with second-degree tears experiencing prolapse, urinary incontinence, and painful sex. Each woman has her own story and requires the right treatment for her own unique circumstances.

Importance of Energy Channels

In Chinese medicine, the channels that energy runs through are called *meridians*. It is along these meridians that acupuncture and acupressure points are found. In Ayurvedic medicine, the "little rivers" of energy are called *nadis*. When we are in radiant health, these nadis are so clear that energy runs through them unobstructed. We feel a glowing warmth and pulsation throughout our body.

As mothers, we are vessels for beings to move from spirit into human form. As a result of being the conduits for this transition, our physical bodies go through profound changes. So do our energetic bodies. Our energy circuitry is shaken when we give birth. Imagine a pan that has layers of residue at the bottom and needs to be soaked for a long time before you can thoroughly clean it. Hot water and soap have to soften the layers before you can scrape them loose. Each of our own inner worlds has some residue. In Indian philosophy, this residue is composed of *samskaras*. Samskaras are lingering past impressions of life events that remain with us, coloring our vision of the present, making us who we are, and creating our temperament.

Samskaras are part of our karmic inheritance, our particular circumstances that we have to negotiate in this lifetime. Rites of passage like pregnancy and birth function like the hot water and soap to soften and loosen all that is hardened in our nadis. All that is calcified into habit and obstructs our ability to truly see, truly know, and truly love can be shaken loose, so we are free to make new choices. This kind of change is not always welcome. We are accustomed to our habits and ways of seeing the world. What is shaken loose is not always what we want to look at, yet ultimately, this rite of passage has the potential to clear the nadis and, as a result, lead us to a deeper sense of freedom and a clearer expression of who we are, in body, mind, and spirit.

Years after giving birth, my midwives told me that I had had a second-degree tear. But when I was receiving bodywork, both my practitioner and I felt that the scar tissue extended into my anal sphincter, which was not severed but had definitely been affected. I couldn't sit well or walk for two months. I was experiencing fecal incontinence, painful sex, and excruciating lower back and pelvic pain. Because the other women I knew who had fourth-degree tears were doing better than I was, I assumed that I must have had a fourth-degree tear also. As I later found out, my body had rejected the suture material used by my midwives to repair the tear. I have low-density connective tissue and had been a vegetarian for twenty years, which I believe contributed to my stitches reopening. Not only did my body naturally have less collagen to form healing bonds in the tissues, but I also wasn't eating mineral- and collagen-rich foods to help support new connective-tissue repair.

It's not surprising that I had difficulty producing enough breast milk to feed my child when so much energy was being taken up by the healing process. My body was recruiting everything it had to repair, and the confusing symptoms only added to my stress levels. Like many women, I had no guide or map to find my way through this territory.

Prolapse

Prolapse happens when the bladder, uterus, or rectum fall below their ideal position in the body, resulting in a feeling of bulging or heaviness (see fig. 31). Women with prolapses say things like "I feel like my insides are falling out," or "It feels like there is something between my legs that wasn't there before," or "I feel like there is an egg sitting in my vagina." The technical term for a bladder prolapse, when the bladder falls down from behind the pubic bone and into the vaginal canal, is *cystocele*. A rectal prolapse, when the rectum is caving toward the back vaginal wall, is called *rectocele*.

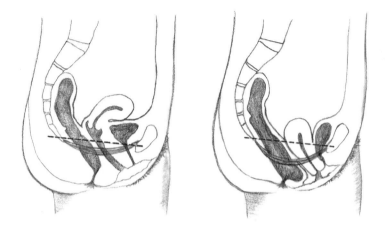

Fig. 31: Prolapse

The following can contribute to prolapse:

- Extended pushing phase in childbirth
- Mechanical delivery (birth assisted by forceps or vacuum extraction)
- Multiple deliveries
- Loose connective tissue/hypermobility
- Premature return to high-impact exercise
- Root energy concerns such as moving, lack of financial stability, lack of tribe or community, family deaths
- Vegetarian diet

While tears are rated in degrees, prolapses are rated in stages. These ratings are relative. The size of each woman's organs and the length of her vaginal canal differ, so there can be a big range between a stage-two and stage-three prolapse. If the organs are slightly below their original position, it is considered a stage-one prolapse. If the organs are lower down with less ligamentous support holding them up, it is a stage-two prolapse. Farther down the canal and visible at the entrance of the vagina is a third-stage prolapse. A fourth stage is when the organs are actually coming out of the vagina.

Why do some people experience prolapse and others don't? There is no easy answer. Statistics show that labor interventions like forceps and vacuum extraction greatly increase the risk of prolapse. We also know that an extended pushing phase as well as pushing with a full bladder contributes to the incidence of prolapse. With each push, all of the organs are pushed downward, and when repeated again and again, it increases the likelihood of their becoming dislocated from their optimal positions. Similarly, women having a second or third child are more likely to experience prolapse. Women who have more elastic, stretchier connective tissue are more likely to prolapse. I also see many women who did not have a prolapse immediately after birth, but they returned to running and intense exercise before their body was ready, which resulted in a prolapse. Avoiding a prolapse is one of the main reasons to stay in bed during the sacred window.

Living with prolapse can be very frustrating. In addition to it being very disconcerting to feel something sliding down from its right place, there seems to be a "two steps forward, one step back" quality to working with it. For many women, it seems like there is no rhyme or reason to the prolapse—one day it's better; the next day it's worse, without being able to trace much of the reason why. Women report feeling better one day on a walk, and then the next day, they are just resting and feel the prolapse lower again, when not even affected by gravity.

All women should know that while they are nursing, their body is still secreting the hormone relaxin, which contributes to looser ligaments. While you are still nursing, be especially patient with your healing process and stay positive about how well your treatment is going. As a strategy to correct prolapse, I recommend you fortify your body first and wait until after you stop nursing before making any decisions about surgery. The statistics for success in surgical repairs for prolapse are not encouraging. It can be very tempting to go the surgical route, especially when symptoms seem like they are not improving or are improving at a snail's pace, but there are no quick fixes for prolapse. That said, a stage-four prolapse, when the organs are outside the body, will require surgery.

Uddiyana bandha kriya, as described in chapter 11, is one of the most effective ways to heal a prolapse. The strong abdominal suction actually lifts the organs up. If you already have experience with inversions, then headstand can be very effective at treating prolapse; combine headstand with uddiyana bandha for a maximal effect.

Community Stories:
Julia

Julia had her third child in Holland, a vaginal birth after two cesareans. She had the help of Kraamzorg, a Dutch system of maternity care that included a nurse who came six hours a day to wash clothes, cook, help with her two older children, and make sure she was resting. After those initial eleven days, Julia's husband went out of town. She was feeling so energized from the help of the nurse and the difference in recovery between the vaginal birth and the cesarean births, that she resumed all her regular activities of cooking, lifting, and taking her kids to and from school. The return to these activities so soon resulted in a second-degree bladder prolapse that she didn't have immediately after birth. Frustrated, she realized that she still needed to rest, and shortly thereafter she sought out holistic pelvic health care.

Women have also had great results with vaginal steaming in working with prolapse. The herbal steam flushes and tones the tissues, increases blood flow, and encourages the organs back upward.

Bleeding after Birth

For the first two to six weeks following birth, your uterus will continue to cleanse itself and you will experience bleeding. The bleeding, called *lochia*, should decrease over time. If you pass a clot larger than your fist in the first few days, you should contact a medical professional. Over the course of your healing, the bleeding will become spotting and will eventually end. If, in that time, the bleeding slows down or stops and then starts again or becomes bright red again, your body is signaling that you are doing too much and need to rest more.

In between when the lochia slows and your period returns, many women have greatly benefited from the practice of vaginal steaming to allow the uterus to be fully cleansed and to create more tone and resiliency in the vaginal tissues.

Eventually your period will return. It is possible to ovulate within six weeks of giving birth, meaning it's possible to start menstruating within two months of giving birth, or to have Irish twins. Yes, even if you are breastfeeding exclusively, you can get pregnant.

The return of a woman's menstrual cycle after having a baby can vary from three months to two years. For women who have experienced birth injuries or birth trauma, periods can be especially painful. Many women experience an exaggeration of symptoms with their period—abdominal muscles feel weaker, pelvic tone feels less accessible, and prolapsed organs feel lower than normal. Periods can feel like mini-births and reactivate the trauma or symptoms that occurred during birth. What can a woman do about this?

Just knowing that this is common can be a relief. Also, if you are trying to heal a prolapse, but you are still nursing and are experiencing heavy or painful periods, be patient. It will take time, but don't lose hope! These shifts allow you to become more attuned with your body, helping you realize how to shift your diet and choice of exercise in order to support the different phases of your cycle.

To this day, I feel a difference in my pelvic-floor tone and organ position between my period and ovulation (follicular phase) and between ovulation and menstruation (luteal phase). When I am in the follicular phase, I am able to do more rigorous exercise and a stronger yoga practice while maintaining a sense of my core. When I am in the luteal phase, I opt for slower, yin-style yoga practice and less intensive workouts, so I feel my pelvic floor and organs are supported. This would be an attuned way for us as women, even those without pelvic-floor problems, to modulate and potentiate our energy throughout our menstrual cycles. Most of us have never been taught to respect the different energies and physical shifts that happen throughout our cycles. Most of us have trained ourselves to be as productive as possible and try to continuously operate at our maximum. When we are young, we feel we can get away with anything, pushing ourselves at every phase of our cycle. But as we get older, imbalances show up more frequently when we fall out of sync with our biology. Giving birth often serves as a deeper awakening to these feminine rhythms, and dealing with birth injuries even more so.

MY OWN MEDICAL REALITY

Postpartum recovery was the first experience in my life that proved to me what I had always believed but had never really felt in my own body—true healing involves all the layers of our human experience—physical, emotional, sexual, relational, and spiritual. One year after giving birth, I returned to the United States to try to get some health care that I understood. Without so much as a pelvic exam but upon hearing about everything I was going through, the doctor I went to told me I needed a full pelvic-floor reconstruction. Since I had chosen a home birth precisely because I valued my own body's ability to birth and heal without intervention, the idea of surgery and more stitching was terrifying to me. I couldn't even fathom exactly what that meant. How do you reconstruct a pelvic floor without creating even more scar tissue? And yet, I had no idea what I *should* do to address all the symptoms and uncomfortable sensations I was experiencing.

I returned to Michele Kreisberg, a holistic pelvic-floor physical therapist whom I had seen before I gave birth. She gave me the first hopeful news: in spite of all my symptoms, I was not the worst case she had ever seen, which was my biggest fear. She believed there was a lot that I could do before pursuing surgery, which was a last resort for me. That visit was the beginning of the journey that resulted in this book.

I threw myself headfirst into figuring out how I was going to get better. I began to suspect that this dearth of information was something that many women must experience. I traveled to Asia to learn about and experience another way of treating postpartum women. I moved to Thailand for four months, where I had access to inexpensive, organic food as well as affordable childcare. I put my daughter in preschool for the first time and invested in thrice-weekly Thai massage treatments at the local hospital. I returned to a meditation practice and a yoga practice made possible by the space created while my daughter was at school. I began to feel relief from my lower back and sacroiliac pain. This is also when I met Ellen Heed, who became my mentor. She was visiting to teach the anatomy portion of a yoga teacher training I was coleading. When I told her about my symptoms, she told me that she was conducting a study on pelvic-floor scar tissue in postpartum women. She asked if I would be willing to be a part of her study, to be documented through photos and videos in exchange for sessions.

It was when I was working with Ellen that I began to see a significant change in the majority of my postpartum symptoms. Our sessions addressed the four domains of pelvic health. Together we were able to form a coherent picture of what exactly was going on. I suspected that the scar tissue was extensive, but with her hands following the paths of every scar, it was no longer a guessing game. We could both feel the path the scars traveled.

In one session, my diastasis knit back together. Normally, diastasis is something that is viewed as requiring intensive and almost constant exercises with splinting through tight belly wrapping. In my case, there was a structural imbalance that, when addressed internally, allowed my connective tissue to reorganize and regain tone. During another session, together with an emotional release, my scar tissue softened and the entrance to my vagina was no longer taut and asymmetrical. Sex became a possibility for me again. I could imagine reengaging sexually.

In my case, the most important quadrants of the four domains of health were emotion and scar tissue. I had experienced a traumatic tear during the birth itself, but the majority of trauma came in the postpartum period, when I did not realize how much support I needed or where or how to get it. That was accompanied by the dissolution of my marriage, and it felt like the ground was falling out from underneath me. So our work together was grieving the loss of the partnership that had created this birth and baby, and grieving the confusing birth scenario that reactivated some core internal wounds, and to do this somatically, by actually feeling the territory where the damage had occurred and lived on as active, self-propagating scar tissue. Biomechanics played a role because of my stretchy connective tissue, made stretchier by years of yoga practice. Biochemistry played a role because my long-term diet was missing meat-based collagen sources, so together with breastfeeding, my body didn't have the key ingredients for repair.

The biggest chunk of my healing was during the work that Ellen and I did together. The next major leap was when I told my daughter's father definitively that our marriage was not going to work out. Knowing that I was ending my chance at the nuclear family I wanted and also that I might be putting my daughter's relationship with him at risk, it was a brave move toward self-sovereignty and profound honesty, with my body leading the way. That night, I felt the two sides of my pelvis slide toward each other, hugging back into my sacrum, and I felt my uterus come back to its normal pre-birth tone. Soon after, when my daughter was two years and four months, I weaned her, and that was another leap forward into more access to my life force.

However, as I mentioned in chapter 4, I was depleted on a deep level. Soon after my daughter stopped breastfeeding, because of repeated monthly sinus infections, I went on a kind of bed rest, taking care of only my most basic needs of food, rest, and work, in addition to mothering a toddler. To rebuild that basic life-force energy required time, patience, dedication, and a lot of faith.

It took me six years to return to radiant health, to the place where any little thing would not send me into a downward spiral of allergies, a cold, or fatigue, and where I had a wider palette of activity choices that felt good to my body. As a yoga practitioner and seeker, I am looking for much more than an absence of pain and mediocrity in the way I feel. Being out of pain is not enough. For me, radiant health is a birthright. Full recovery from my daughter's birth required that I call everything into question about the way that I had structured myself, my identity as a woman, partner, daughter, and mother. It also required me to live what I had been teaching—that true healing requires attention to the interconnected nature of all the layers of who we are.

Know that healing is available to you too. Use this model of the four essential domains of health to get clearer about what is happening in your body, mind, and spirit that is contributing to how you are feeling. I know how hard it is to prioritize your own health when there is so much to take care of and adjust to just day to day. It is every new mother's dilemma. When we are in the motherbaby unit, it can be hard to even peek our head above water to have perspective and recognize what is going on. With this model, you can simplify what may seem like an overwhelming situation and reach out to get the support you need.

SUMMARY

- There are four essential domains of health that need to be considered when trying to heal any symptom, including a birth injury—biomechanical, biochemical, emotions, and scar tissue.
- Birth injuries are a potential outcome of giving birth, but they are not inevitable nor are they permanent. Healing without surgery is possible in most cases.
- Incontinence is common but not normal. It's not always caused by weak muscles. It can also be caused by hyper-toned muscles or scar tissue.
- We must be our own advocates for our pelvic health because medical professionals are not always informed about postpartum birth injuries.

Reflections

- Before having a baby, which quadrant of the four essential domains of health was the most stable and healthy for you?
- Before having a baby, which quadrant was the one that called your attention most often?
- Do you have insights on any vulnerabilities that you may have carried into birth that are now contributing to your postpartum healing process?

Practices

- If you have a birth injury, make your own pie chart with the four essential domains of health. In your estimation, what percentage of your symptoms are due to biomechanical, biochemical, emotional, or scar-tissue causes?
- Now that you have a pie chart, you have a better sense of the care you need and the direction to go for your care.
- If your symptoms are mostly emotion- and trauma-related, the best place to start is body-based therapy.

- If your symptoms are mostly biomechanical, the best place to start is physical therapy or holistic pelvic care.
- If your symptoms are mostly biochemical, the best place to start is a naturopathic doctor or holistic nutritionist.
- If your symptoms are scar-tissue related, bodywork and the home protocols, like castor oil packs, vaginal steaming, and self-massage, are your best direction.
- Most likely, your symptoms are a combination of the four. It's hard to see ourselves clearly, so if you have pursued one of these avenues and it hasn't worked, you may need an outside eye to help you with your assessment, such as a STREAM practitioner.

··· 9 ···

owning your birth experience

Most of us think of birth as a rite of passage, and it is, but what we don't realize is that birth is just one of many rites of passage that make up the process of becoming a mother. And to understand our postpartum experience, we also have to understand our birthing experience. For many of us, that means reclaiming our place as the protagonist in our own narrative.

Birth is a reckoning, no matter how it goes. Whether your birth is a scheduled C-section or an unassisted home birth, it is a unique journey. Birth changes us in ways that we may recognize right away or that may take years to recognize and assimilate. It also affects our relationships to our babies and to our partners. How our birth goes affects how we traverse the rest of our motherhood journey, how we see ourselves as women, daughters, mothers, and partners.

In our modern world, where there are few formal rites of passage, birth and becoming a mother is a distinct one, changing both how we view ourselves as women and how society views us.

THE PASSAGE INTO MOTHERHOOD

The term *rites of passage* was coined in 1961 by Arnold van Gennep, a Dutch anthropologist who studied the way that people all over the world acknowledged life transitions, from birth to death. For a complete rite of passage, he identified three phases common to all rites of passage: separation, transition, and incorporation. This means that a person separates from a previous world; occupies an intermediate, transitional space; and then becomes part of a new world.

I am indebted to midwife Rachelle Garcia Seliga, creator of INNATE Postpartum Care trainings for birth and health-care professionals, for her profound insights and synthesis of the map of rites of passage and motherhood. In traditional societies, the changes were as much internal processes of the psyche and soul as they were physical, geographical processes of reshaping and relocation. People moved locations and changed dwellings based on their phase of life. For example, a pregnant woman would leave her family hut, go to a hut where pregnant women and new mothers lived, and then, after a few months to a few years, would move into a new dwelling in the family area. In modern India and Japan, many women still leave their husbands' houses; return to their own family homes where their mothers, aunties, and unmarried sisters live; and then after six weeks or so, they go back to living in their married homes. Women made an actual physical move that represented the transition. Expressions like "crossing a threshold" or "going through a portal" described literal passages. Today these are metaphorical phrases but they are actually journeys that all women experience, whether or not there is an external physical acknowledgment of it.

Separation

The first phase of the rite of passage, separation, can sometimes even be described as a death. In the motherhood journey, this first phase of separation is pregnancy. While our culture views pregnancy as a time of ripening and blossoming, which it is, there is simultaneously a distancing from our previous identity. Becoming pregnant, when we become a home for another being, we leave behind our individual, autonomous self and our maidenhood. We leave behind membership in the world of nonparents. When we become pregnant, who we were starts to fall away, giving way to something new.

Transition

After a period of separation, we move into an intermediate, transitory space. We've let go of one thing and haven't moved into the next. We don't belong to our old group; we are not our old selves. But we don't yet belong to a new group, and we don't know who we are yet becoming. We are being born into a new version of ourselves. In the transitional space, a person doesn't have a specific place or identity. We are in a suspended space.

This transition phase is often the most dramatic and the most colorful phase, requiring a seemingly superhuman feat. The transition is the vision quest, the journey to the top of the mountain, the first solo hunt or fasting. In this phase, the body is the ritual site of sacrifice. The ego is dismantled; we come into contact with something larger than ourselves. We have to dig deeper to find resources that we didn't know that we had. We face the unknown. We're pushed to our physical, mental, and spiritual limits. Our soul is tested.

In the motherhood rite, the transition phase is birth itself.

Childbirth is the gateway for our babies to move from the inner world to the outer world. For most women, giving birth is a pronounced encounter with our deepest reserves that we may not have even known were there. We are the vessel to bring spirit into form. Childbirth is the gateway for our baby to move from the inner world to the outer world. Birth is a part of a transition into a new self-understanding, a new physical self and a new social self, which we will continue to integrate through the last phase.

Incorporation

The final stage is called *incorporation* or integration. The word *incorporation* comes from the Latin root *incorporare*, meaning to "unite into one body," "embody," or "include." After the transition phase, a person returns to her community with wisdom, lessons, experiences, and physical marks from her journey. She is welcomed into the community and encouraged to share the fruits of her experiences, so everyone can reap the spiritual benefit of her journey. She eventually becomes part of the new social group.

This phase of integration in a woman's rite of passage into motherhood is the postpartum period. Many women are shocked by the postpartum experience because they were focused on getting through the birth, as if the birth were the ending. Birth is an ending, but it is not *the* ending. Birth is the beginning of a longer transitional period, a process that is different in length and tone for every woman. There is another level of ego death and grieving over the separation from her pregnant self and birthing self. The pregnancy is over. The birth is over. Another level of mothering has begun.

A rite of passage is not a linear path. The rite of passage of motherhood is a series of concentric circles and spirals. Pregnancy itself has the three phases of separation, transition, and integration, and being in labor has these phases as well. Qualities of each phase may be present throughout our transition to motherhood. We may disintegrate and reintegrate at various points of the journey. A rite of passage is also an individual experience, as much as it is a universal one. Each person will find different stages of the journey to be more challenging or more rewarding.

YOUR RITE OF PASSAGE

The questions below can simply be done in your mind, as a reflection, or they can be answered in a journal entry. Either way, try to truly stop and consider your answers to these questions, as opposed to just reading the questions as quickly as you can.

- In what new ways did you meet or are you still meeting new parts of yourself during your pregnancy, birth, or postpartum experience?
- How do you see these three phases of separation, transition, and incorporation in your pregnancy experience? How is it for you without your pregnant belly?

- Which parts of the rite of passage of pregnancy were or are most significant for you? What were the turning points for you during pregnancy when you had a glimpse of what you were letting go of or who you were becoming?
- What parts of you have you let go of through this journey?
- What parts of you are you fiercely holding on to?
- If you had to tell a pregnant woman one thing that you learned from your birth experience, what would it be?

Your Community and Rites of Passage

This rite of passage is a profound gift and invitation to experience life in its fullest expressions. As women, we are made for this experience. For centuries, indigenous peoples have created rites of passage for boys as they become men, putting them through grueling tests so they could feel what they were really capable of. Men had to fabricate experiences to put the ego on the chopping block, and to imprint a relationship with the natural world. As women, we don't have to create rites of passages for ourselves. They are built-in, as we cycle with nature, living the life/death/life cycle every month. Biology constructed our very existence to include rites of passage, of which motherhood is a major one.

In times past, there were intermediaries facilitating the journey through a rite of passage. Elders would facilitate the changing of conditions and guard against disruptions from the outside, so the person experiencing the rite of passage could stay fully immersed, free from distraction or outside interference. Each phase had its own specific preparations, reverence, and support, and received its due acknowledgment. When people return from their quest and are neither recognized for their triumph nor able to share their gifts with their community, they experience isolation and confusion, as if their journey made no sense or does not have value. They feel as though they have lost their path. When a person receives recognition, support, and a place to share her experience, she will emerge on the other side stronger, more resilient, and with a deeper sense of self—everything a new mother needs.

While we may not be able to orchestrate a community reception for our emergent-mother self, we can and must claim the power of our experience. As women, we must recognize and appreciate, not minimize or normalize, the power of this rite. We must express ourselves for our community to hear. We must take up space so that our community can receive and value our gifts received through our mother rites. This begins with mining our birth story for its gems and meanings. From there, rather than simply sharing facts, details, and outcomes, we can share the truths and revelations of our experience.

MINING THE BIRTH LESSONS

On that crisp winter day in Rio, as the sun began to set, I was aware that I was laboring alone. An animal marking its territory, I traversed my apartment, pacing, at least ten times over. My body led me around, making a map of the space where I would soon birth a baby. Everything seemed to be going according to plan. My midwife had arrived in the morning and set up the tub, the plastic sheets, and everything needed for the labor and delivery. She had sent my parents out for the day and night, as we had discussed. My mom had really wanted to stay, but the midwife encouraged me to minimize the number of people at the birth to reduce potential confusion. My husband didn't speak English. My mom didn't speak Portuguese. I didn't know what I'd be speaking during labor. My midwife spoke decent English, but we had done all our appointments in Portuguese. We'd call my parents when the baby was born.

My husband came back from lunch and fell asleep after having a beer. My midwife was napping. What was going on? Didn't anyone care that I was having a baby? After forty-two weeks and four days,

I was finally in labor, but where was everyone? Why was I doing it alone? Why wasn't anyone there with me?

I'd been laboring for twelve hours, what's often described as "early labor"; there is a gradual climb of intensity. I never went through the "bake muffins and plant in your garden" zone of early labor, where you're supposed to go on with your life as usual. From the minute labor began, it had required my full attention and presence. I was already in primal territory, not caring that I couldn't see without my glasses or that I was naked.

My midwife returned, saw my face, and immediately said, "I'm sorry I abandoned you."

But it was too late. I'd already made a pact with my daughter that it was she and I against the world. Forget about everyone else—she and I were going to do this birth together. From that moment on, we were ensconced in an insulated bubble together that no one could really get into. Our safety depended only on each other—on my body, my will, my determination, and her strength.

To this day, I continue to be awed by the ways that the dynamics that occurred during my daughter's birth continue to play out in our lives all these years later. We are a tight, interdependent dyad, and any attempt at slackening the umbilical cord is deeply felt on both of our ends. While I did invoke a pantheon of deities as I chanted the entire labor, the deeper message was not to trust in the universe and the women who were present. The message was that the two of us better stick together if we wanted to make it. Our survival depended not on a deep and interconnected family unit, not on the support of known and familiar earth, not on an endless net of birthing mothers and birthing women and midwives for time eternal, but on the unbreakable bond between the two of us.

Each new mom has a birth story. And whether we're interested in sharing it with everyone or don't want to really go over the details with anyone else, it's important that you accept, explore, and own your story. Below, we explore ways to do that.

Community Stories:
Tiffany

....

I worked with Tiffany via Skype. At three weeks postpartum, she was feeling very unsettled and a bit desperate. She had just given birth to her second baby at a birth center in the water with her midwife and partner by her side. A Feldenkrais movement teacher, she had imagined following her own body's cues and impulses to love and dance her baby into the world. Feldenkrais is a method of moving the body in non-habitual ways, many of which imitate stages of developmental movement, so that we find the most efficient ways to move, which creates less pain and more freedom in the body. The system itself is concerned with naturalness, which was definitely one of her values. She described kissing her husband as she labored, the idyllic golden lighting in the room, and how she felt in control and powerful. She explained how her baby emerged, perfect, into the water. And yet, there was one moment that she kept replaying over and over again and she couldn't get it out of her head.

There was a moment when she was on all fours, hands on the side of the tub, deep in labor and beginning the pushing stage. The midwife told her that if she wanted to give birth in the tub, she would need to flip onto her back, because the midwife didn't want to risk the baby being born in the air and then slipping into the water. Tiffany did not want to be on her back, but did want to have her baby in the water. Everything was happening so fast, the thought passed through her head, *Maybe I'd rather get out of the tub altogether*, but it didn't make it all the way into a request.

So she obeyed and turned onto her back. In defaulting to the midwife's authority at that moment, she lost the thread of connection to her deep intuition, her body, and her truth. Her daughter was born soon after, and interwoven with her joy was a sense of confusion. That feeling remained until we were able to pinpoint the source of her unrest, the place where the internal matrix had been torn, and stitch it back together. She was finally able to say out loud that she would have preferred to stay on all fours, even if that meant getting out of the bath and departing from her original wish to birth in the tub. To any outsider, it would have looked like Tiffany had the ideal birth—in the water, like she had wanted to, with a healthy baby girl. But Tiffany had left behind a piece of herself that she needed to go back and retrieve so she could fully inhabit her body in the present moment and relax into mothering.

In our work together, she was able to pinpoint that moment as a place of skipped communication between her and her midwife. She was disturbed that she didn't know of the limitation of that position beforehand. And in the throes of transitional labor, she submitted to her midwive's authority. Afterward, she needed to be on her hands and knees (in our session work) to complete the process and open up a space for her to experience having a choice.

Narrating Your Birth Story

Telling the story of one's own birth experience is a way to unveil the meanings within. Unconnected events and anecdotes are experiences without meaning, and when we don't look deeper, we cannot always fully mature and move forward. Connecting fragmented memories and unearthing a coherent narrative is part of the process of returning to wholeness after birth, and in an experiment led by Italian researchers Paola Di Blasio and Chiara Ionio (see below), making connections has even been proven to decrease postpartum depression. The potent insights we get from our memories can increase our emotional and spiritual growth and, in many cases, empower us to move forward and imagine ourselves and our lives in new ways.

Our dominant cultural narrative is that, as long as mother and baby survive the birth experience and are relatively healthy by Western medicine standards, the birth was successful. This discounts many women's experiences—even though, yes, they are healthy, and yes, their baby is healthy, their bodies, minds, and souls are still deeply affected. Like so much of the way our culture works, the process itself is exchanged for the outcome, in this case the birth experience is discounted because you have a healthy baby. You see this all the time in the way we talk about birth with each other.

"How was the birth?" a friend asks.

And the answer is "C-section" or "unmedicated natural birth."

If someone is going to summit Mount Everest, their experience is much more elaborate than if they made it to the top and back. For the climber, there are several vivid and critical moments that define the experience much more than simply "I summited" or "We didn't make the summit." While giving birth, there are pivotal moments when we face ourselves at deeper levels, when we come face-to-face with unexpected obstacles or unanticipated reservoirs of strength. When we reduce the experience to the outcome—and specifically to the rote idea that as long as a woman is alive, everything went well—we overlook an untapped resource. The woman and the community miss out on a chance to gain wisdom and maturity from her experience.

Here are the exact directions given to the women in the Italian study:

Once the door of your room is closed, write [down] for ten to fifteen minutes continuously, without lifting your pen from the paper, the thoughts and feelings that you had during labor and delivery. It is important for us that you describe also your most secret feelings and thoughts which you have not told, nor would tell, to anyone.

It is essential that you let yourself go and come into contact with your deepest emotions and thoughts. In other words, write what happened, how you lived through this experience, and how you feel about it. Everything you write will remain strictly confidential.

Consider doing this exercise yourself. With the relatively short time limit, you also might find yourself more motivated to start the process of writing about the birth. For some women, giving voice to their experiences is not easy, but it is a powerful process in which you have the chance to become the protagonist of your own story.

The research showed that the most effective decrease in postpartum anxiety or depression symptoms came when women wrote out their unfiltered story within forty-eight hours of the birth experience. However, there is no time limit on making meaning of one of the most powerful and significant experiences of your life. Wherever you are in your recovery process, take the opportunity now to write your story. Even if you have written it out before, it's worth it to write it out again to see what, if anything, has changed.

Even though we've talked a lot about making meaning out of the story, when you sit down to write, free your mind of this intention. Take a few deep breaths—as many as you need to feel your thoughts begin to slow down. As you contemplate your birth experience, notice how your body feels. Decide to write your story from your heart, paying attention to the sensations in your body. If you are right-handed, place your left hand on your heart as you write to remind you to feel your body. If you write from your mind, you will feel pressure to get the order of events and a coherent narrative right. It is your story, so you can include any details you want to. But notice if you are struggling to remember what came first and what came last, rather than how you were feeling during those moments. It is not important to remember every detail in perfect order. It is important to document significant moments and how you were feeling during them.

Community Stories:
Michaela

When Michaela came to see me, she had just become pregnant for the third time. She was experiencing a surge of unresolved feelings from her first two pregnancies. Her first birth had been an unnecessary cesarean. She had just arrived in a new country with totally different birth practices than she imagined. After laboring for what she thought was a relatively short time, she was told that she was not progressing and needed a cesarean. Without being able to communicate well in a foreign language, she kept trying to advocate for herself but it wasn't working. Generally confused about what was happening, she ended up delivering her baby through a cesarean. The memory of that delivery had haunted her but she had been able to move past it, she thought, by returning to her home country and putting some space between herself, her family, and her birth experience.

Her second pregnancy had unexpectedly dredged up some of those old unpleasant and negative feelings she remembered from after her first birth, but ended suddenly in a miscarriage. When she became pregnant for the third time, instead of feeling the elation she expected, the floodgates of the grief from the first two pregnancies opened. Plagued by sadness and doubt, she came to see me.

A very proper and polite woman, she had a hard time communicating her true feelings about the poor care she had received during her first birth. She apologized several times and often physically covered her mouth when she spoke. She was trying to protect the reputation of her doctor, worried that I would think she was blaming and badmouthing her doctor if she shared her real thoughts. After I assured her that our session was confidential and that I wouldn't judge her doctor, she was able to express her true feelings. Through tears, she shared the words that she had tried to say. She explained asking for more time, but being told that there was no more time. She explained that she asked if there was something wrong with her baby, and deducted there wasn't because no one was rushing in to help. She felt that because they took their time, they were just wearing her down until she finally gave in to the outcome that was easiest for them.

When she allowed herself to express her frustration at not getting straight answers and her anger at the confusing situation as well as with the nurses and doctors, and also recognize the ways that she had been a warrior by challenging the birth staff at multiple moments along the journey, she found forgiveness for herself for giving in to a cesarean, recognizing that she had expended all of her resources for struggling in such a complex situation. When she allowed herself to tell her story without worrying about what I would think about her or what anyone would think of her, she was able to appreciate her own experience and imagine different outcomes for her upcoming birth. She made the courageous choice to change doctors and set herself up for the kind of birth she knew she wanted to have.

When I saw Michaela several months later, she had gained the courage to change health providers. She chose a birth team that was supportive of VBAC—a vaginal birth after cesarean. We had discussed in session how important it was for her to learn to express her emotions, of all kinds, without caring so much about how her feelings were perceived by others, and she shared that she had been having some more frank conversations with her family.

The next time I heard from Michaela, she wrote to tell me that she did indeed have the redemptive birth experience—a VBAC—she so hoped for with a doctor who listened to her.

Other Ways to Tell Your Story

There are many ways to tell a birth story. Although there is specific research on the benefits of writing it down, artistic expression of any kind can be a way to work through the story in the body and through creative channels that can often lead us to different, possibly unexpected meanings. Some women may like to paint, draw, make a collage, or even make a voice recording.

Instead of or in addition to writing, you can speak it aloud and record it, or make art with it. Here are some ideas:

1. With one hand on your heart or on your womb, take several deep breaths. Clear your mind and begin to reflect on your birth experience. Without pressure to write in a correct chronological sequence, write down the moments that stand out as you look back on the whole experience.

2. Record your birth story. Tell your story and record it as a voice memo on your phone.

3. Use colored pencils or pastels. Recall some of the turning point moments of your birth. You don't have to label those turning points positive or negative. Keeping that one moment in mind, allow your hand to move across the page. Draw that moment. You don't have to be a good artist to do this. You can even close your eyes while doing it so that you don't expect it to be accurate.

Whenever you do it, there will be power in telling your birth narrative. You may find critical pieces of self-understanding and understanding of your mother-child bond or your partner bond in the process. You may find that the ways you look at yourself are influenced by specific statements or circumstances from the birth.

Stories don't always have wonderful endings like Michaela's. But it is a common occurrence when I work with women who are having difficulty conceiving, that when we dig into the birth experiences they've had, including abortions and miscarriages, we clear a pathway to understanding and meaning about what happened in their bodies and in their psyches—and they often then conceive. Contrarily, when women haven't learned how to truly own their birth experiences, they often unconsciously end up with the same kind of care they received the first time, even if they make a concerted effort not to. I've seen women who were 100 percent clear that the care they received during their first birth was substandard and, in some cases, inhumane, turn around and repeat the scenario again the next time. It is often the births where something needs healing whose narratives especially need to be told.

TENDING TO A BIRTH THAT NEEDS HEALING

When we say the words *birth trauma*, most of us think of babies and what they go through in birth. But mothers are experiencing one of the most transformative experiences of their lives when they give birth, and birth is getting more complicated than it has ever been. Women are inundated with choices from start to finish in their pregnancies—the frequency of ultrasounds, whether or not to vaccinate, where to birth, which birth classes to take, even how to breathe. While most women make the choices they feel will allow them to have the best birth experience possible, no one can control or know exactly how birth will go. Women often suffer in silence, not noticing their new pains or limitations, as they are focused on their babies and families. If they do realize how they feel, they don't know where to turn.

Trauma is not defined by an experience itself; it is not the event that happened. Trauma is determined by our body's ability to metabolize an experience. Something that is traumatic for one person may not be disturbing for another. More important than why this happens, which may be the coalescence of our personal, familial, and cultural history, is how we recognize it and what we can do about it. To be human is to experience trauma. Fortunately, to be human is also to experience healing.

The Nature of Trauma

So why do some women experience trauma while others don't? In *Birth in Four Cultures*, Brigitte Jordan explains that there are three primary factors that determine a woman's sense of satisfaction about her birth experience:

- her perception of control;
- how supportive she found the birth environment and the people in it; and
- her prior vulnerabilities including her own birth and childhood, prior abortions or birth experiences, and her history with depression.

Even the most prepared woman, one who has chosen every part of her birth scenario as well as her support team and has done healing work on her own past, may experience a birth that registers as trauma. Trauma is a loaded word, but it is not a life sentence.

In Michaela's story, the lingering imprint of trauma was caused by not feeling in control at that specific moment during her birth. Her body recalled and reexperienced a feeling of helplessness when in that particular physical position. The position sent her body into a mild freeze, and she didn't have full access to her voice. You can see how delicate this situation is, given that, overall, Michaela was in control and in a supportive environment.

Birth itself is a vulnerable act. We are usually naked, exposed, and fully open in the most intimate part of our body. Our neurochemistry heightens our sensory awareness. In giving birth, we feel and sense more. This affects and influences our memory. As a result, subtle behaviors and position changes can strongly influence a woman's internal experience.

Birth injuries are physical injuries that occur during childbirth, as described in chapter 7. If you have never heard of the term *birth injuries*, you are not alone. Geraldine Barrett et al. found that over 80 percent of women in the United States emerge from childbirth with some kind of pelvic scar tissue, and the CDC reports that over 30 percent of women deliver babies via C-section, which is major abdominal surgery. Women who experience birth injuries are more likely to experience birth trauma and PTSD.

Birth trauma and birth injuries are more frequent than we realize. Between 25 and 34 percent of women report that their children's births were traumatic, even though the staff and their support team may not perceive it that way. Birth trauma includes more than just danger of death to mother or baby; it also includes physical injuries and the perception of danger, as well as feelings of extreme fear, aloneness, disrespect, lack of control, or helplessness. When we only think of a major catastrophe, death, or accident as trauma, the smaller but also significant, undigested pieces are left untreated and dismissed altogether. In doing so, women may blame themselves for an inability to move on or to feel satisfied about a birth that everyone else thinks went great. (See the section "Cross-Training Your Nervous System" in chapter 4.)

In the case of a birth that needs healing, writing out a birth story can potentially cause more harm than good. If you notice that your heart accelerates or you start to feel anxious or frantic when considering returning to the events of the birth, then this is not the time to revisit your entire birth experience. Instead you can work with your experience in other ways.

Recall if there is one moment when you felt helpless or over-powered. While there may be more than one moment, see if you can choose just one. This is important—you can't work with every moment at once. If it is not immediately obvious what moment that is, then choose the first moment in the experience that you remember feeling out of control.

RENEGOTIATING A BIRTH THAT NEEDS HEALING

1. Choose ONE moment in your birth experience when you felt helpless, overpowered, or out of control.
2. If you feel a very high level of activation (recall this from "Cross-Training Your Nervous System" in chapter 4 and also check in with yourself to see if intuitively this feels helpful) when recalling this moment, start with your powerful imagination. Visualize what you would have liked to have happened. Imagine what you would like to have said, how you would like to have moved, possibly who you would have liked to have with you at the time. See the whole scene in your mind the way that you would have liked that moment to have gone.
3. If the level of activation feels medium, write down the answers to the same questions as above: What you would like to have said, how would you have liked to have moved, or who would you have liked to have with you at the time?
4. Now that you have imagined or written about how you would have liked to react, speak, move, or respond in that moment, notice how you feel in your body. Stay with this practice of noticing for at least thirty seconds.
5. Then let your eyes wander around the room and notice things that catch your eye. Where do your eyes land? Notice what happens in your body and your breath. As you orient back into the room you're in, become more present in the here and now.

It is very important that you not skip to rewriting your entire birth story the way you wish it would have happened. This is not about denying the circumstances of the birth you had or living in fantasy. This is about giving your nervous system a chance, in small pieces, to complete a cycle of self-protection and agency that may have been thwarted during the birth. The nervous system is sensitive and responsive, so working with one moment at a time is the appropriate pace for a birth that needs healing. You might not feel an immediate change, nevertheless respect a slow pace in working with sensitive material. If this process is appealing to you and also effective, then you may be compelled to renegotiate more than one moment. If you decide to work on more than one moment, leave a day or so in between, so that you have a chance to process the changes.

If at any moment, this process feels like too much, return to the rule of threes (from "Cross-Training Your Nervous System"). Sometimes it is necessary to have a trained professional that you can develop trust with guide you through this process of renegotiating the birth events.

If you experienced a traumatic birth, seek out the help of someone who is a trained counselor and versed in working with women and trauma. Birth Story Medicine, the work of Pam England, is a powerful modality for processing birth material; it is led by women practitioners who are specifically trained to help women find the medicine, the healing gems, in their birth stories. I also recommend working with a Somatic Experiencing practitioner who can work with the physiological patterns in your body, possibly utilizing touch. Birth is a visceral experience and also a sexual experience. Because birth and sex happen through the body, deep healing often happens by including touch and the body in the process of coming to resolution and closure of the birth experience.

I wish there were a better word to use than *trauma* to discuss these issues. *Trauma* is a word that people tend to either under-identify or overidentify with. It becomes a label that we cling to or reject.

The truth is that we have all experienced trauma in life. Not one of us moves through life perfectly able to process and digest every circumstance and event that comes our way. That unprocessed or undigested material gets stuck in our system. Afterward, we are on autopilot, often repeating thoughts or behaviors that we may not even notice have been ingrained from the experience. Many women realize that their birth experience was traumatic for them because they cannot stop thinking about what happened and continue to feel the emotion of it. Many other women experience postpartum depression or anxiety, major shifts in their self-image, sexuality, or relationship, and don't realize that it is related to something that happened during the birth experience.

Whatever the outward circumstances of your birth were, if there are still parts of your birth experience that haunt you, that you find yourself going over and over, that just don't sit right with you, make sure you do the exercises in this chapter. They will help you begin to own your own birth experience. Beyond that, please give yourself the relief of seeking out a professional, whether therapist, midwife, or postpartum doula to help you. Trying to just get over it won't work without looking more deeply, and sometimes that requires the support of a wise person who knows something about birth and can help you understand your experience.

ACCEPTING THAT YOU ARE NOT WHO YOU WERE

Women are often surprised by the "negative" emotions of grief, feeling overwhelmed, and sadness that they experience in a time when they expected to be supremely joyful. As a society, we tend to glorify the intoxicating feelings of having a baby, so when the darker emotions come, they can be unexpected and upsetting. Whether it is a loss of her carefree self, the loss of her relationship before the baby, or the loss of her big, pregnant belly, the feelings of grief are real, and almost all women feel them. When women can be honest

Community Stories:
Leslie

Leslie came to work with me after she gave birth for a second time. Her second delivery was a cesarean, and she wanted to know if it was going to be possible for her to try for a vaginal delivery when she got pregnant again. She was worried about scar tissue on her cervix that she felt had impeded her delivery, made it unable for her to dilate fully, and had been the cause for the cesarean. Her doctor had tried to break up the scar tissue during delivery but not to great enough effect. Leslie became flooded with emotion as she told me about her first delivery, when the scar tissue had developed. In her second trimester of pregnancy, she learned that her baby was no longer alive, and she decided to deliver that baby vaginally. Of course, she was heartbroken but had come to terms with the spiritual significance of that baby in her and her husband's life. When we began to work with her second birth story, she realized that her body did not open because she associated that dilation with birthing a baby that was not alive. Her body was protecting her from having that experience again. So rather than feeling safe and open to dilate, she remained safely closed and delivered a healthy baby girl via cesarean.

Highly engaged in her own process and quite uninhibited, she touched her own cervix, feeling the scar tissue. Her own manual work along with mine, together with the understanding of the unconscious belief that was operating during the birth, has led her to feel confident that both her body and mind will allow her to have the natural birth she wants when she decides to have another baby.

with themselves about their true feelings, without layering on shame or guilt for not feeling how they think they should, they can relax knowing that it is the natural process of becoming a mother. They can gain greater access to the full experience of mothering and life—in all its shades and textures.

These emotions are gifts that allow us to experience more of the depth of who we are. Most of these emotions are neither desired nor comfortable, yet they can be the grist for our evolution. Exploring them can give us clues as to how we can resolve patterns of behavior and emotion, changing them not only for ourselves, but also for our children.

I emerged from the birth of my daughter with one reinforced core belief and one new, imprinted one. The core belief was: I am alone in the world and I have to do everything myself. The new one was: It's me and my daughter against the world. They have each had their own repercussions.

Under stress, these beliefs become default operating systems, unconscious internal mantras. When I'm conscious and awake, I work with them, recognizing when they arise and opting for behavior that gives my system information to the contrary. When I am in the "I have to do everything myself" mode, I pause and get in touch with my own internal little girl who feels stranded and overwhelmed and ask her what she needs. Usually she just needs to be heard. Then I look realistically at my life and take inventory: Who is on my side? Who is there to help me? I take a moment to express gratitude for that support—my parents, my daughter's schoolteacher, my landlord, my sister, my clients, and my friends. Then, if I still feel like I need help, I reach out and practice humility while asking for what I need.

It's hard to know what comes first sometimes—the belief or the reality. For my daughter and me, this core operating system that says our survival depends on our coalescence as a united front has meant that we have mostly lived in one-bedroom or studio apartments, without spaces of our own. We have lived on three different continents sharing the same room and same bed. Men have come and gone from our lives, and what has remained is the two of us, each the major pillar for the other. I have many times mistaken codependence for interdependence. And I am divided when she tells me that I am the one person in the world that really gets her. Part of me thinks there is so much beauty in our closeness and trust. The other part wants her to feel safe and understood in multiple arenas by many sources. Both are true. I do what I can to reinforce a feeling that she is supported by many pillars, not the least of which is life itself. Yet I see how that birth pact, where I placed will above life, permeates our reality to this day. We are both living into the understanding that we are drafting on the waves of the flow of life.

Each birth has its own intricacies and lessons for each mother that are hers to discover over time. This is why it's important to tell your story your way. It's okay if things didn't go as planned. It's okay if they did but you weren't as ecstatic about them as you thought you would be.

Even if things did go as planned and you and your baby are both "fine," there will be things—emotions, physical sensations, and so on—that you won't be prepared to deal with immediately. It will help you feel more whole and emotionally healthy if you process them in your own time. How your birth experience goes affects your postpartum period. When women feel disappointed, discouraged, or traumatized, digesting the experience can be extremely challenging. It takes time and support.

SUMMARY

- Birth is one part of an extended rite of passage that is the transition to motherhood.
- Telling your birth story is an important part of coming through birth in one piece, and it can even diminish symptoms of postpartum anxiety and depression.

- It is okay and even normal to have "negative" feelings after a birth.
- Some births are traumatic for mothers, even if they may have not been life-threatening, or appeared to be so from the outside. Working through the birth trauma can be the key to physical, emotional, and spiritual healing.

Reflections

- What parts of yourself have you met through the rite of passage that is birth?
- Is there a part of your birth experience that is lingering with you that you continue to think about or wish would have gone differently? How do you feel about each member of your support team during your birth experience? How do you feel about your partner when you think about the birth? How do you feel about your relationship to your baby when you consider the birth?
- Can you identify a core belief that was activated during your pregnancy or birth experience? Can you identify a new core belief that arose out of your birth experience? Identify a core belief that was activated during your pregnancy, birth, or postpartum experience. (That may be something like "I am alone," or "I can't trust people in authority to listen to me.")

Practices

- Write, record, or draw out your birth experience.
- Choose one moment in your birth story that won't leave your mind. Recall that image and visualize what you would have liked to have happened. Imagine what you would like to have said, how you would like to have moved, possibly who you would have liked to have with you at the time. See the whole scene in your mind the way that you would have liked that moment to have gone. Then notice how you feel in your body as you imagine that new scene.

··· 10 ···

deepening intimacy

Having a baby changes everything—our bodies, our self-images, and our identities as women are never the same, so it is no wonder that our relationships change as well. Most new parents are wary about how their intimate relationship will change when two becomes three—or three becomes four, and so on. Some gloss over it with a "we'll figure it out; how hard can it be?" attitude. Others worry and troubleshoot, anticipating the worst. Our cultural dialogue basically straddles these extremes of denial or devastation as well. Men are warned that their sex lives will be over and their wives won't so much as notice them anymore. Women are told to endure sex even when they don't want it or when it's painful, to keep the relationship going. Everyone ends up fearing and anticipating how their relationships, and specifically their intimate lives, will weather becoming parents.

During this time, we are all redefining and rediscovering who we are, so we have the chance to clarify our roles and figure out how we want to move forward. Much like the deeper layers of physical, mental, and emotional patterns that are revealed during the immediate postpartum period, relationship dynamics are also unveiled at a deeper level. Just as women are often thrown consciously or unconsciously into remembering their relationships with their own mothers as they question how they themselves will mother, which is explored more in chapter 13, men too are revisiting their own relationships to parenting.

Becoming a mother and becoming a father are distinctly different experiences, both important and significant.

After having a baby, our roles as partners change, so we need to be aware and accept that the ways we look at each other may change. There is often a natural return to more traditional gender roles. For many women it can feel like a demotion or a loss of power. Even though empathy and nurturing, the feminine traits that are activated in early motherhood, are enormously valuable, most of us haven't learned to value them equally with productivity and intellectual prowess. The gravitation toward more stereotypical gender roles makes most women cringe, so deep has been our commitment to equality, but biology tends to rule at this time.

The Swahili *mamatoto* (motherbaby) and Gutman's invention of *mommybaby* or *babymommy* (not *daddybaby*), indicates the unique and specific role of the mother at this time. The survival of the newborn depends on the interconnection with the mother. In the fourth trimester, a mother can do things for a baby that a father cannot do. What a man can do at this time is protect the sacred window and provide what the motherbaby needs.

Partners have to adjust to each other in these new, changing roles. A new level of effort, contact, and willingness is required. What once may have been automatic now begs for our attention. Because relationship satisfaction determines so much of our overall life satisfaction, it is worth this attention and effort. Also, our children benefit from thriving, connected, and loving parental connection.

When relationship experts Doctors John and Julie Gottman studied relationships headed toward separation or divorce, they found that, in a high percentage of couples, the beginning of the deterioration of their relationship began during the year after their first child. In the first three years after a child is born, marital satisfaction typically dropped 67 percent.

Thankfully, the Gottmans continued their research to find that radical decline in relationship satisfaction was not a foregone conclusion.

They studied the 33 percent whose relationships did not suffer from the transition to parenting and found that, with preparation, forethought, and skillful communication, relationships could weather the radical change set in motion by becoming parents. Many of these tools are included in the "Safeguarding Your Relationship Postpartum" section of chapter 3. The fact that you are reading this book already puts you at an advantage when navigating this change. Acknowledging that this is a significant change, exploring expectations of yourself and each other, having a plan, and enlisting adequate resources are all part of what will protect your relationship. This phase of life has the possibility to strengthen your intimate relationship, deepen your shared foundation, and create the platform for joyful parenting.

MAKING SPACE FOR PARTNERSHIP

It is so easy for all of our focus to go to our new babies. They require so much of us. Their needs and routines are changing so fast, and there are so many logistics to manage. In the midst of shifting and adjusting, if we are not mindful and before we know it, all we're talking about with our partner is what size diapers we need and what we're going to eat for our next meal.

Additionally, we are flooded by hormones that encourage bonding and nesting with our babies. Oftentimes, women feel so nurtured by the close connection to their babies and also so overwhelmed by the demands of a newborn that touching their partner falls to a low place on their list of priorities. This can cause partners to feel overshadowed and undervalued. And thus begins a dynamic that creates distance and resentment. As your partnership is the cornerstone of the health of the family, it deserves care. Keeping lines of communication open about how you are doing, how you are feeling, and what this process is like for you is critical to staying connected to each other and to the relationship.

Remember that your partner is your greatest untapped resource. As often as you can, come back to remembering that you are on the same side, that you are a team. All the rest, good food, and massages in the world will most likely not compensate for feeling disconnected from, angry at, or hurt by your partner. You want to proactively work

How to Create and Maintain Closeness with Your Partner

Start with friendliness and an attitude of deep care. Choose kindness even when you are frustrated, sad, or discouraged. Prioritize unconditional positive regard for one another, knowing that you are on the same team.

1. Acknowledge each other when you come in and out of the room with words, eye contact, a nod, or a wink. Take care not to rush past each other. Look up from your devices to acknowledge each other.
2. Hug each other until you feel "the drop," (see "Hugging" on page 233) that is, until you feel each other settle, your bodies soften and melt in, your breath slowing.
3. Speak in a low, soothing tone. Notice when you are talking fast or loud. Take a deep breath. Commit to communicating calmly when possible.
4. Check in upon waking up and going to sleep. This can be as simple as saying your partner's name and "good morning" or "good night."
5. Pay special attention to separations and reunions. Say "hello" and "goodbye" with eye contact. If needed, repeat when you will be seeing each other again, what time you will be home, and how you will connect during the separation (texting, e-mails, phone calls, or maybe you will be out of reach).

to create what Stan Tatkin, the relationship innovator and author of *Wired for Love*, calls a "couple bubble." A couple bubble describes a mutual agreement that your partner is your highest priority, that you share things with him or her before anyone else, that you return to the bubble as your core source of security, and that you commit to maintaining the clarity and sanctity of the relationship between the two of you. Visit or revisit the "Couple Bubble" exercise in chapter 3.

As long as you are working to create healthy bonding and attachment with your baby, why not extend that to your partner as well? It's simpler than you might think, focusing on the little things, like eye contact and acknowledging each other as you come and go in and out of the room, or in and out of the house.

Recognizing the well-being of the relationship and your partner as a priority is a crucial first step and foundation to maintaining that bond. Dedicating time most days to connect with each other is the next. A once-a-week date night is the popularized way of dedicating time to your relationship. It's a great idea, but somewhat unrealistic and maybe even undesirable for the first three months post-birth. What's more important is maintaining the thread of connection in your day-to-day interactions, so you aren't just waiting for that time once a week to catch up on everything.

With this foundation of loving-kindness and ongoing connection, it is also strengthening to spend three to five minutes a day in contact. Initiating this requires only willingness, not turn-on or desire. Willingness to spend time in the ways outlined below, whether gazing, breathing, or touching, will further deepen the foundation of your relationship and the sense that you can rely on it for support. These three to five minutes of contact aren't to review to-do lists; they are to simply be together. A few minutes of nonverbal contact is a consistent, manageable step toward connection with each other. While it may seem clumsy at first, set a timer and just do it. It may become one of your favorite parts of the day. Make the effort to keep your partner connection at the center, and not allow all eyes to literally turn to the baby.

There are many ways to connect, and you might try out a few of these suggestions to see what you and your partner enjoy the most. We tend to think of connection as something that either does or doesn't happen, and we are not sure why. Like learning to play a musical instrument, ongoing connection takes practice. Every day that we practice is different, and we can start to appreciate how varied and layered our experiences are.

EYE GAZING

Eye gazing is a way to connect and feel each other without having to talk. Set a timer for three minutes. Get comfortable standing, sitting, or lying down, and simply look at one another. It seems so simple, but it is profound. You may notice that emotions arise. Your eyes may well with tears. You may laugh in joy or embarrassment. You may get bored or frustrated. You may find yourself closing your eyes or looking away. Resist the temptation to talk. Continue to look in your partner's eyes. Invite relaxation in your body and in your face as you do so. At the end of three minutes, acknowledge your partner with a bow, a nod of your head, or a hug. Say thank you.

SYNCHRONIZED BREATHING

In a comfortable position—sitting, standing, or lying down—place a hand on your partner's heart. Have him or her place a hand on your heart (see fig. 32). Feel your hand move as your partner breathes. For several breath cycles, just notice the rhythm of your partner's breath. Maybe you will feel the beat of his or her heart. Is the breath fast or slow? Is each breath similar, or is each one changing? Your hand is there to notice and receive this information, not to do anything with it. Your partner is also noticing your breath. You may notice that without even trying to sync up your breaths, you start to fall into rhythm with each other. Without talking, there will be a dance of who is leading and who is following. Whose breath should slow down? Whose should speed up? Who will meet whom? It's a dance of following and leading. The goal is not to be perfect and sync exactly. The goal is to be in unspoken dialogue, feeling and listening to each other's bodies.

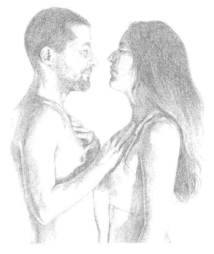

Fig. 32: Synchronized breathing

HUGGING

....

A full-body embrace is a wonderful way for partners to calm each other. When we hug consciously, feeling the contact of our bodies, after a minute or two, there is usually a distinct settling in. I call that moment "the drop." Hormonally, the drop is when your body releases the hormone oxytocin, a love and bonding hormone that counteracts the stress hormone cortisol. You will feel your mind and thoughts start to slow down, and you will be able to sink into the sensations in your body, really feeling them. As you settle into your own body, often you can feel the drop in your partner also. Your partner's body lets go of a layer of tension and leans into you, almost molding to your body. You might even hear a contented sigh. Commit to hugging until you both feel the drop, and then stay for a minute or two, enjoying that higher level of presence, attunement, and bonding.

APPRECIATIONS

The purpose of this exercise is for partners to focus on and remember what they love about their other half. During a time that can be full of questions and even anxiety, it is easy to get pulled into only seeing what's wrong. When our inner state is shifting in a way we have never experienced, we often look around for explanations. Many women direct their anxiety toward their partner. This is a chance to listen to one another and reconnect with what has worked and what is working in your relationship. You can start your sentence with something like "One thing I love about you is _____." "One thing I am so thankful for about you is _____." "I want to express my appreciation to you for _____." This practice can take as little as one minute.

If there is something that is bothering you, I recommend the following practice of open listening so that each person is able to really talk about what is happening for him or her. Speak in "I" statements. Avoid blaming your partner. Communicate about how you are feeling and what that's like for you.

OPEN LISTENING

The objective of this exercise is for each person to have a chance to express her- or himself. As the speaker, you can talk about whatever is on your mind. The intention is to clear the air and give voice to what is keeping you from connecting in the present moment. Unlike the previous exercises that focus on connection, this exercise focuses on freedom of expression without editing and is helpful if you are feeling stuck and resistant to the earlier exercises involving touch.

Choose one person as the speaker and one as the listener. Sit side by side with opposite shoulders touching, looking away from each other. Since you are not looking at each other, you have a chance to express yourself without being influenced by how the other is reacting, reading their facial expressions and body language. Also, this helps you practice how to listen and consider another's point of view. We practice listening without interrupting. Listen with open awareness and curiosity about your partner's experience. Practice empathizing with your partner's point of view. What does the world look like through his or her eyes? Here are some things for both of you to remember while listening:

- Do not interrupt. You will both get a turn to speak, so don't interrupt to "correct" or interject with your perspective.
- Avoid sighing or shifting your weight in reaction to your partner's sharing.
- Suspend your own story and your own version. Take time to really hear your partner's point of view.

When one person is done speaking, trade roles. Your share does not have to relate to their share. This is a time to speak from your heart about yourself and your own experience. This is not a time to prove anyone right or wrong. After you have each had your turn, turn to face each other. Take three deep breaths together and complete the experience either by thanking each other or continuing the conversation.

Your Partner's Birth Story

In chapter 9, you processed the birth story from your point of view. Now it's time to share your experience with your partner and hear your partner's experience. It's important to talk openly about each person's experience of the birth, celebrating successes and airing lingering confusion or resentments. The birth process can be the glue that brings partners together or a wedge that drives them apart. The intensity of birth creates a unique hormonal configuration that alters the way memory works. In "birth land," time is not linear. There will be moments that we don't remember at all or that we cannot place in sequence. There will be moments that are forever etched in our bodies and minds. In any case, memory is never totally accurate and is highly influenced by our past experiences. We don't usually choose what does and doesn't stick with us.

Therefore, when your partner shares his or her experience of the birth, you may be surprised to hear a version that is different from yours. Your partner may have memories of moments you don't recall at all. What seemed important to you may not have seemed at all important to him. What is important is listening to each other without arguing over the details. Listen for the moments that are turning points. Listen for the places that your partner repeats him- or herself, gets emphatic, or changes the volume of his or her voice as clues to what may have been exhilarating or scary for them.

You remember from my birth story that I labored alone for some time. I had prepared for and planned a home birth, and my daughter's father had been part of that process. Yet when he saw me in labor, he panicked and reverted to his conditioning that hospitals were the safest place for births. When I saw how scared he was so early on in labor, I knew that I couldn't count on him to advocate for the least intervention possible in whatever scenario I ended up in, which was my wish. I knew that my labor was only going to get much more intense over time.

His panicked state also made the labor environment tense, so my midwives began a process of trying to divert and distract him. He remained in another room in our apartment until the moment that my daughter was actually coming out, when I yelled for him. To this day, the birth is an experience that evokes grief for him. He felt alienated and unprepared. He wanted to be there to support me but was confused about what was normal. He was not pacified or relieved in the least to be sent out for lunch or relegated to another room. He didn't feel like anyone was there to orient him. He lay in the other room listening to my sounds intensify from moans to screams, wondering if I was okay and questioning his place. He ended up separate and helpless.

We had our first conversation about the birth in the middle of the night about eight weeks after our daughter was born. It was a deeply connected and healing moment for both of us. I listened to his experience, to his version of the birth of his daughter. He listened to my version of the experience, and without any need to change, fix, or convince, we simply cried together at what both of us knew was one of the most intense and formative experiences of our lives. We see each other infrequently now, but when we do, it is not uncommon for the birth to come up.

LISTENING TO YOUR PARTNER'S STORY

Use your listening skills from the "Open Listening" exercise, but this time face each other. Ask your partner about his or her experience during the birth. What was easy for your partner? What was hard? What was surprising? Then stop asking questions, and just listen. Give your partner time and space to express him- or herself. This is time to listen to what happened for your partner during the birth—the story he or she tells has wisdom and keys in it.

Oftentimes, it takes a couple of rounds of telling our stories over time to find the meaning they have for us. We may feel confounded by something that our partner is hanging on to that felt insignificant for us. Our partner may not understand why we cannot move past or get over parts of the birth that seemed necessary, normal, and even practical to them. We don't actually have to understand. We just need to listen wholeheartedly.

Our stories evolve over time and that is healthy. When a narrative never changes, we are not growing or developing our ability to see the meaning of our stories in deepening layers. With an experience as big as giving birth and becoming parents, it may take time to find a way forward with a joint narrative that honors each other's experiences and to make the repairs necessary for healing.

Once a week, carve out twenty to thirty minutes to have a more extensive check-in that combines some of these tools. It's helpful to have a structure to check-ins, especially if things have gotten difficult or charged. While it can seem a bit unromantic, having a roadmap to fall back on eliminates anxiety knowing that both of you will be able to check in and be heard. Tend the burning embers and commit to finding each other. This is the foundation of returning to a sexual life together.

FULL CONNECT

1. Sit close to one another, making eye contact for a minute or so.
2. Hug until you feel the "drop."
3. Share one appreciation of your partner, and receive one appreciation.
4. Check in:
   - How are you doing?
   - How am I doing?
   - How are we doing?
   - How are we doing as parents?
   - How are we doing as a couple?

5. Close by holding each other or sharing another appreciation.

Following these steps allows you to remember who you are as individuals, and that you are indeed having individual experiences. Becoming a mother and becoming a father are different journeys. This process allows you to honor and hear about these differences and also reminds you that you are a team. There exists an "us" outside of your baby or your children.

Keeping the channels of communication smooth and open goes a long way toward easing anxiety, deepening connection, and smoothing out the road back to sexual intimacy (more on this topic in chapter 12). The communication tools outlined above help you to stay current with each other. There is so much flux from hour to hour, day to day, and week to week in new parenting that keeping up with each other and how you are doing in the midst of these changes takes some ninja-level attention. All the effort is worth it when you realize that your partner is your biggest ally.

Worlds open when you are able to meet each other in the ever-evolving present moment. While the stereotype is that men want sex all the time, the Gottmans found that postpartum what men were really looking for was attention from their partners. With so much attention focused on the baby, men felt invisible. They needed to know that their wives still found them attractive and desirable.

Community Stories:
Ruthie

"I was a changed person. How can someone be intimate with someone who has changed completely, someone who is even unrecognizable? I transformed. My needs changed—logistically, emotionally, physically, sexually. I felt so different inside on every level. I wanted to explain it to him, but it was so hard to. Sometimes I wondered if he understood at all that a changed woman was sitting next to him, or if he thought it was still the old me? How could I feel intimate with someone who wasn't at least trying to understand how I changed? How could I explain it to him if I didn't understand it myself? I think this just requires presence and patience and respect, and loosening our expectations of each other. It requires an openness to a new life. Sometimes we longed for our pre-baby relationship. Those dynamics, the ease and freedom and the comfortableness that we found together. Suddenly that relationship was gone, and we were in unknown territory. The baby's birth called us to mature in general. The baby gave us motivation to invoke our more mature selves so that he would have parents who are in love and treat each other well."

WRITE A LETTER TO YOUR PARTNER

From where you are right now, from the changed woman that you are, from how you feel this moment, write a letter to your partner. (If you are single, write a letter to yourself about this new person that you are and what you need.) Tell your partner what you need him to know. Tell him how you are feeling about your body, your emotions, your family, your relationship, and whatever else feels important. Encourage your partner to write you a letter as the new dad or partner or man they are now. Below are two examples that might be jumping-off points for you or serve as inspiration to start your own letter anew.

To My Partner (from a New Mom):

- I am experiencing so many things on so many levels I can barely express how it all feels.
- If I am crying, there might not be anything wrong. I might not know why I'm crying. Just hold me and tell me it's all going to be okay, even if you don't know what "it" is.
- The more space you can give me to not have to return to being the person you used to know, and being willing to get to know me as I am each day now, the more space I will have to show myself to you.
- I actually do need your touch right now.
- Please tell me that I am doing a good job. No matter how confident I might seem, I am always wondering inside if I am doing a good enough job at mothering. I need reassurance.
- The more you pamper and care for me now, the faster I will be whole again, and filled with gratitude for how well you cared for me in one of the most vulnerable times in my life.
- I still want you. I feel like a virgin. I am not sure who I am sexually. I want to explore, and it may mean doing things differently than we did before. I hope it will be better.

Your partner may also want to write to you. If you share the chapters of intimacy and sexuality, it will help your partner understand that you are both going through identity shifts with some common themes. The knowledge that the postpartum period is a very unique time will help to give the perspective that this is a tunnel you are moving through and there will be a new reality on the other side. Here is an example of a starting point or some inspiration.

To My Partner (from a New Dad):

- Take my hand and lead me back to your body in a way that feels good to you.
- You are so in love with this new being we created. The baby needs you so much. You are doing an amazing job. I need you to see me too.
- I don't know what to do when you talk about how dissatisfied you are with your body. I love your body.
- I love talking to you, but I need it not to be all about logistics and to-do lists.
- It's okay if you want a pause from sex for a while, but I still need to know that you find me attractive.
- I know that I don't do things the way you as a mother do. Please respect me as father. I will find my own way. It will be different than yours. Eventually that will be a good thing.
- Give me the benefit of the doubt.
- Show me how we can connect in a way that feels good to you.

SUMMARY

- Though studies show that relationships are drastically changed by a birth, they can change for the better with care and communication.
- Plan for the changes to your relationship and its roles with your partner and be open to discussing them now, in the postpartum time.
- Consider that intimacy is about communication and understanding, not just sex, and focus on building that as opposed to worrying about jumping back into PIV sex.

Tenderness, honesty and clear communication are the foundation of this pivotal time of transition from couple to family, or smaller family to bigger family. Some of these practices are helpful all the time, but why not use this time of great opening and possibility to rededicate yourself to the values that you want to be the foundation of your family? The love that is awakened in your heart for your baby can also be radiated inward toward yourself and outward toward your partner. In the face of the normal challenges of decision-making and exhaustion, your partner bond can become the battery pack that recharges you.

Reflections

- Notice which of the connection exercises seems easiest. Write about what this exercise reminds you of and why it is most appealing. What would you hope to gain from the experience? How would you want to feel after?
- Notice which of the connection exercises seems difficult and maybe even a bit cringe-worthy. Write about what seems difficult, and what you might feel if you were able to get past resistance and give it a try.

Practices

- Commit to maintaining intimacy and practice one of the connecting exercises—eye gazing, breathing, hugging, or appreciations.
- Listen to your partner share his or her experience of your birth story.
- Write your partner a letter as the New Mom and the New Dad that you are now.

Creating a Postpartum Ritual

Just as a mother blessing or baby shower is a way of gathering support for the passage to motherhood, a postpartum gathering is a powerful way to celebrate the end of the fourth trimester. This ritual can open the door to the outside world, marking the passage from an inward focus on strengthening a woman's family bonds, and her immune and nervous systems, to a slow introduction to the external environment. Of course, a woman's transition to motherhood has no finite deadline. In many ways, the end of the fourth trimester marks just a beginning of a woman's return to an individual sense of self. Many women return to work some time from two months to four months. It might be supportive to schedule this blessing to coincide with your return to work.

A postpartum gathering might look like this: Supportive women and mothers gather together in the new mother's home. These women bring nourishing food, flowers, candles, a poem or story to share. They come prepared to form a sacred circle of protection around the mother and ready to hear her birth story, as well as her reflections on what she has had to leave behind to arrive where she is. While listening, the women might bead a necklace or a bracelet, draw a portrait, take photos or simply sit in openhearted silence. After hearing a story, other mothers may share a story about their experience of this new motherhood territory—to offer their unique medicine. This event represents the crystallization of the departure from the maiden and arrival into the seat of the mother.

Part Three

BEYOND THE
FOURTH TRIMESTER

.... ❧ ....

THE UNFOLDING LAP

I AM MOTHER whose entitlement unlocks the doorless room
The home of a mystery that flays the soul's skin
Carving ego and rendering the oily mind into light.

I AM MOTHER who grows dreams in my belly
From my blood drinks the Tree of Life
Rooted in heaven until the birth quake
Splits me open in revelation and relief
And I awake from the nightmare of separation.

I AM MOTHER carrier of the secret told since the beginning
Hearth of the future, unfolding lap, volcanic breast
A daughter of uncertainty, the crone's executrix
The ultimate harvester of hope.

I AM MOTHER so hear me! Listen with labyrinthine ears
To the purpose of sound, sense the movement of your cells,
And the pulsing message from your bones that resonate with this;
Serve the Breath-Maker and be the BirthKeeper the Earth needs now.
Your mother will be so proud.

—JEANNINE PARVATI BAKER

Now, you're past your fourth trimester, which means the major hormonal and physical adjustments may be behind you, but your transition to motherhood continues. While we, of course, realize that mothering is a lifelong journey, it's not often stated that the changes to our physical and sexual identities will continue. Just as the changes our bodies and psyches go through during puberty take years to get used to and integrate, so too will the changes after giving birth continue.

But this shouldn't be something that frightens or deters you. Your identity as a woman and a mother will continue to evolve, and opportunities for growth and transformation abound. While no one can predict the direction of your own personal journey, there are some tools that will help as you prepare for it. Befriending and rediscovering your body—through exercise and sex—and discovering your individual mothering style are steps in the right direction.

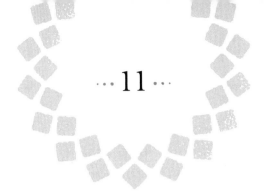

··· 11 ···

rediscovering your body

Nurturing and growing a baby in your womb, and then giving birth, requires massive restructuring of your body. And though you had ten months (if you carried your baby to full term) to get used to mainly incremental changes in your posture, weight, center of gravity, and so on, the cumulative effect of pregnancy and birth is dramatic and takes time to get used to. Even if you don't suffer from a tear or a prolapse or didn't give birth via C-section, or experience any of the other "traumas," your body has still just gone through a staggering amount of change. It's important that you return to exercise and your sexuality in thoughtful and informed ways, so you can continue to pursue the physical things you enjoy for the rest of your life. You'll want to give yourself some time, and some tools, to reacquaint yourself with your body, while being open to changes and respecting and even learning to love the new body you have.

LOVING YOUR BODY

The postpartum time is an invitation for us to reevaluate our relationship to ourselves in almost every way. The patterns of how we relate to ourselves, how we relate to our families, and how we relate to our partners come to the surface. What we may have ignored earlier arrives as an unannounced guest, allowing us the possibility to choose a different way, and potentially even heal elements of those relationships.

Our relationship to our body is a primary one, and it is foundational to how we orient in life. We will inhabit this body until we die, so if we can befriend it, rather than judging, berating, and fighting with it, we only stand to sweeten our lives. Learning to love our changing, evolving bodies may be one of the most worthwhile, albeit difficult, processes we will ever engage in as women. Loving our bodies, in the midst of objectification, pressure, and judgment is not just a personal victory but also a radical act of embracing maturity and wisdom.

Judging ourselves harshly isn't just a personal problem. Whole industries exist, predicated on our unhappiness and dissatisfaction with how we look. The beauty and cosmetics industries and pharmaceutical companies benefit from selling us the idea that we need to buy things to look better and take drugs to feel better. One standard body type—tall and very thin—is upheld as the ideal, while we know that we are born in all shapes, sizes, and proportions. Models and most actresses represent a beauty standard that glorifies youth and a boyish shape. Photoshop erases what are considered to be imperfections and reshapes bodies in service to this narrow ideal of perfection.

Meanwhile, our bodies as mothers who have recently given birth have full breasts, round and sagging bellies, and generous thighs. The absence, not the presence, of these feminine or motherly or womanly features that are inherent to giving birth are what defines models and what we are taught to believe is beautiful. Yes, what is upheld as our cultural standard of female beauty is narrow hips and flat stomachs—the exact opposite of what a new mother has. If we look outside ourselves to define our beauty, most of us can't win. Indeed almost everything is stacked against us inhabiting our full magnificence whatever our shape or size is. Therefore it is a radical, revolutionary, personal, and political act to live in harmony with our female bodies.

The changing nature of a pregnant and post-birth body is an invitation into a new or deepening relationship with loving-kindness and impermanence. When we go within, with curiosity, there is a ripening treasure trove of wisdom to be gained by accompanying the changes and learning to love ourselves just as we are.

The first step is to move away from comparing ourselves to how we used to be or how we want to be and steady ourselves in the present moment. Our body and its form is in continuous evolution throughout our lives, it is just more noticeable and dramatic than ever after giving birth. To approach this process with patience and kindness is to offer ourselves the possibility of delighting in the changes, however odd, unexpected, and possibly even unwelcome, rather than simply bearing them.

After the momentous event of carrying life and giving birth, the body takes time—almost universally, it's longer than we'd like it to be—to reassemble itself into its new shape. Comparing ourselves to actresses that are back to work three weeks postpartum or to our friends who got back into their prepregnancy jeans in two months, only causes us to suffer. We are once again called to have long-term vision and perspective so that we are not tempted to abuse ourselves by crash dieting or overexercising in an attempt to manage anxiety or insist that our body look a certain way outside that it may not be ready to support from the inside.

The second step is to shift our focus from judging and evaluating how our body looks to expressing gratitude for what our body has been through and what our body has done. This shift is a mindfulness practice.

FROM JUDGMENT TO GRATITUDE

1. When you hear your inner critic piping up to make a negative comment about your body, be vigilant. Be mindful not to spin into a criticism of the criticism. Pause and take a breath.

2. Remind yourself that you are in the middle of a monumental process that is probably longer than you anticipated that it would be. Remember that where you are right now is not where you will be forever. Say to yourself internally, "I just grew and birthed life and am still nurturing that life."

3. Then choose to remember a part of your body that you love or one thing that you are grateful for about your body. Touch that part of your body, name the appreciation out loud, or write it down.

The next step is to understand that how our body looks has nothing to do with our ability to experience pleasure. Most of us mistakenly think that if we were in better shape or if we had a flatter stomach or if we had a different whatever, then we would feel better about ourselves. We think that if our body would change in the way we wanted it to, we would be happier or more content or feel sexier. The good news is that there are no physical prerequisites for happiness or our ability to experience pleasure. We can be happy, content, and sexy right now with the bodies we have. Imagine the power we can generate when we do not depend on looking a certain way to have access to our joy and pleasure!

The foundation for everything in the rest of this chapter and whole section of this book is patience, loving-kindness, and refined listening. As you return to bigger activities like exercise and sex, do so with the utmost care and kindness. There is no race to win, no rush. You can always stop, and begin again.

REDISCOVERING YOUR BODY THROUGH EXERCISE

The truth is that after ten months of pregnancy, the birth itself, and nine months of car seats, baby carriers, stroller attachments, and feedings, every woman's body could use some structural realignment. Many women take the approach that they will just wait until they have all their kids and then deal with their body. But it will be much easier for you to maintain a sense of comfort and well-being in your body, which means a return to comfortable exercise and sex, if you take care of it as you move through your motherhood journey.

The hope is that at the end of your lie-in time—the infamous six-week mark—you schedule a visit to have your pelvic floor checked out by a pelvic-floor physical therapist, so you can do any necessary core repair work needed. If you are already past your fourth trimester and haven't seen a pelvic floor specialist, you can still do so.

At this time you can also consider deep-tissue massage to work through some of the knots and tension in your upper back and between your shoulders from bending over, carrying car seats, and nursing. I love Thai massage, but take care not to be stretched too far. Because flexibility is so prized, yoga teachers and Thai massage practitioners often get excited and assist in deepening flexibility when they see the opportunity. Make sure that you make it known that you want to work on stabilization more than pushing the edges of your flexibility.

Nine months postpartum is an ideal time for a postural overhaul. Rather than trying to spot-correct specific knots or discomforts, this is a wise time to invest in modalities that take into consideration the body's whole structure and the interrelationships between the parts of the body.

Two excellent modalities for this holistic approach are Structural Integration and the work of Moshé Feldenkrais. Structural Integration, also known as Rolfing, works with the connective tissue to help return optimal posture to the body with a once-a-week session for ten weeks called the "Ten Series" or "the Recipe." Functional Integration, one part of the work of Feldenkrais, is a hands-on movement reeducation process that allows the body to return to more optimal balance and function. Both modalities result in less pain and easier posture so that you can use your body the way you want to. It's possible to become even more upright and stronger than before you had a baby.

Learning to Exercise Safely

After you've rested for the first six weeks and incorporated core breathing and gentle movement, you may feel ready to return to something more active. This is the time to take gentle walks, preferably on a flat surface, for about fifteen minutes or so.

Walking outside in nature is optimal. But if that is not available, then an elliptical machine is the next best choice. I recommend placing your hands on your head, rather than leaning on the railing while walking on the elliptical so you have a true gauge of your balance, and internal stabilization is a requirement.

Remember, this is a time to gradually build your stamina, taking into account all that your body has gone through. Of course, we all get impatient to return to the things we love doing, but keep in mind that being conservative now will help you recover more fully and return to activity without regressing. The trend toward more intense and aggressive exercise is everywhere. Every new exercise trend that arises is something more challenging. As far as I am concerned, *new mom* and *boot camp* have no business being in the same sentence.

Swimming is fabulous at this time, especially kicking. Laps with a kickboard can help strengthen the tiny muscles in the pelvis alongside your tailbone and sacrum—the stabilizers you will need when you return to your normal movement routine. Swimming with a kickboard also places you in a mini backbend that is the exact opposite position to the one that you find yourself in as you gaze down at your baby and bend over a lot. Experiencing less gravity also helps to lift weight off the pelvic floor, which can be a relief for anyone who is feeling heaviness or discomfort when standing or walking.

I recommend waiting until at least six months postpartum to return to exercise that includes running or jumping. In the meantime, what I see most often in my practice are women who come to me at six months postpartum because their backs are killing them. They started running or rigorous yoga or CrossFit six weeks postpartum and their structure just couldn't support it. Then they have to do reparative work and deal with the overburdened muscles in their back that compensated for the lack of pelvic-floor and abdominal-core support earlier. This is why it's necessary to drill in the importance of waiting to go back to such vigorous activity. You don't have to go through this frustrating, unnecessary, and longer process of returning to optimal function! Take things slow and easy, and rest!

It is a great idea to continue the foundational core-strengthening exercises from chapter 7. We need to strengthen the inner muscles first, before working with activities that make demands from the larger muscle groups. Now is a good time to start a deeper practice of activating and lifting your core muscles, and yoga offers the age-old tool of *bandhas*.

Bandhas for Healing

The yogic practices called bandhas, or energetic seals, have been instrumental in my healing process, as well as the healing process of many of my clients. Practicing them can provide tremendous relief after so many months of heaviness and downward weight in the pelvis. They can relieve low back pain and regulate digestion as well as possibly help to prevent or restore prolapse, depending on its root cause.

Recently a form of exercise has emerged called *hypopressives*, which was developed in Spain and is just making its way to North America, to address conditions like prolapse. There are some graphic YouTube videos showing women's genital anatomy while doing hypopressives to show that it is effective in lifting the organs. Hypopressive practice is an elaboration of uddiyana bandha kriya, which literally means the "flying uplock cleansing," a yogic technique of massage and lifting the organs. Think of it as an antigravity move for your internal organs.

Get ready for a little weirdness, and don't do this practice if you are still bleeding, have your period, or are pregnant. In those cases, you want to allow for downward energy, not try to reverse it and lift it up. The practice of bandhas can begin around the six-week mark. It is also important that you have practiced the breath for length, as well as the week-by-week movement practices (outlined in chapter 7), so you have mobility and are able to breathe into your ribcage. The practice is only effective when the ribcage can lift, so the organs have some place to go.

UDDIYANA BANDHA KRIYA

1. From a standing position, inhale into your chest.
2. As you exhale, arch your back and place your hands on your thighs as your knees naturally bend.
3. At the end of your exhale, hold your breath and round your spine like a Halloween cat (see fig. 33).
4. Plug your nose with one hand and take a false inhale. (That means breathe in with your nose plugged, so you won't take any air in, which will create a vacuum seal that sucks your organs up.)
5. Hold your breath as long as feels reasonably comfortable.
6. Release the suction and let your belly go, and then breathe in again normally.

Like anything, this takes practice. Over time, the suction will get increasingly strong, and you will feel layers of your belly and your pelvic floor being pulled up. You might feel a bit of suction at your throat too. That's normal.

The next stage is to add *mula bandha*, the "root lock," which we might consider the yogic version of a Kegel. Mula bandha is more than just a physical action, but physical actions can help to ignite this subtle, yet powerful energy in the pelvis. For women, mula bandha is described at two different locations. Some texts describe it as residing in the perineum, the skin between the vaginal opening and the anus. Others describe mula bandha as the mouth of the cervix in women. I think they are both right and describe the necessity for awareness in these two levels of the pelvic floor.

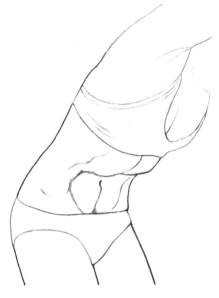

Fig. 33: Uddiyana bandha kriya

After you have practiced uddiyana bandha kriya, you will notice that there is less downward pressure on your pelvic floor. This is an optimal opportunity to be able to engage your pelvic-floor muscles. Please note that visualization is an important step in every action. Imagination activates neural pathways and is the first step to action, especially to a new and unfamiliar action. Eventually it is important to get confirmation about whether these imagined actions are becoming manifested actions. There are two tiers of actions, and they can be practiced independently or together.

The first one is to pull the four corners of your pelvic floor together as if tightening a drawstring. To feel if the drawstring action is actually happening, you can roll up a washcloth and place it lengthwise between your sitting bones. When you exhale and activate the drawstring action, you should feel your sit bones getting closer together, compressing the washcloth a bit. The other movement is to pull the vaginal walls in and lift them up, together with the cervix. This is a small movement, so millimeters of movement are what we are looking for.

PELVIC-FLOOR IMAGERY

Here are some cues and images that might help spark your brain and wake up your pelvic-floor muscles. Try them out and see if there is one that speaks clearly to your body.

- Imagine that there is a ladybug at the entrance of your vagina. Imagine you have a tissue and you want to pick up the ladybug without crushing it. With an exhale, feel the walls of your vagina scoop around the ladybug and lift it gently up.
- Imagine that you have a lover inside of you. On an exhale, hug your lover in tighter, squeezing him closer.
- Link the center of your pelvic floor and the center of the crown of your head together in your imagination. Imagine a thread between them. On an exhale, feel the thread being pulled skyward, and feel your pelvic floor lift along with it.

If you aren't sure whether your imagination is linking up with actual actions, then external feedback is incredibly helpful in confirming that your effort is converting into strengthening and activation in your pelvic floor. This is sensitive territory, as you may not feel ready for penetration yet. Please do listen to your body, and if penetration of any kind feels like too much, then wait. If penetration sounds okay, the best means of feedback are your own fingers, a yoni egg, a dildo, or a lover—in order of intensity. If you place two fingers inside your vagina and then separate your fingers while squeezing, you will be able to feel if your vaginal walls hug your fingers back toward each other. With a yoni egg—a crystal or jade egg that you insert in your vagina—you can feel whether your muscles are able to hold the egg in and if you are able to lift it up inside a bit. Most women will need the biggest size of jade egg to work with as the muscles return to normal tone. If it falls out right away sitting up, start lying down.

A dildo will cover a broader surface area, so you will have more to squeeze against, which can feel more satisfying. A bit more complex, depending on how you look at it, is enlisting a male partner to help you. This can be a bit charged if you are feeling self-conscious, and you also need him to stay still while you practice squeezing him. Penetrative sex itself can be helpful, provided that you feel ready for it on all levels. You may have never tried to do any of these movements or you may have done them before and are mystified about why they are so hard now. Patience and persistence are needed.

You might want to find a teacher, physical therapist, or sexological bodyworker who can help you. These practices are also most effective in combination with an internal pelvic-floor checkup to make sure that your brain is coordinated with your pelvic muscles. Sometimes we think we are using them, but we're not. To make your effort most effective, it's affirming to have some external feedback about what is working and what's not. Connection to these muscles will help you to feel anchored, directed, and confident.

This can all sound very clinical, but talking about the pelvic floor is talking about the most intimate part of our body. Most women have a difficult time even finding language that feels comfortable— not too clinical, not too embarrassing, but still accurate. Our healing often depends on getting literally reacquainted with our experience of our sexuality in our body. Our intimate anatomy may not look or feel familiar to us. In sidling up to this sensitive and perceptive area, we stay open to the currents of life, to our creative energy, and to the possibility of receiving our partner again.

RETURNING HOME TO YOURSELF

Our sexuality is our own. Each of us has a unique way that we have constructed ourselves as sexual beings. We have personal, familial, and cultural scripts that have taught us and continue to influence how we relate to our body and to sex. We have life experiences imprinted in our minds and bodies, informing us about what is safe, what is acceptable, and what is desirable. Our culture is filled with ideas about what is and is not sexy. Even defining sex is not that straightforward. When most people use the word sex, they are referring to what is known as PIV penetration.

The postpartum time calls us home to ourselves, to our relationships to our own bodies and our sexuality. For many women, this is hard to even consider. We are so conditioned to please; there is so much pressure to satisfy others and to place our needs or wants after others', that it is new territory to claim our bodies and our sex as our own. Sovereign sexuality can be foreign territory. In the lifespan of a woman, the transition to motherhood is one invitation to place our needs first when it comes to sex.

Because our body feels so different in the weeks, months, and even years after having a baby, we need to connect with our bodies in these changes. Instead of demanding that our body perform, behave, or act like it used to, we must listen to our new body and what her new needs are.

We have explored how to take care of our bodies with rest, food, exercise, and bodywork. Now we turn to taking care of our sexual selves. It's common for women to feel aversion toward looking at their own genitals after giving birth. Some women have never looked at their own vulvas or vaginas before, so they don't have a visual reference point, but they still feel like things aren't right or are out of place. When women do look, they often feel that everything down there looks different.

As has been discussed earlier, for many women, their vulvas and vaginas *are* different than they were before. Some women sustain birth injuries that require stitching and repair. Some women's proportions have changed—where their labia are or what is visible from their vaginal openings changes. Some women have skin flaps or tags that weren't there before. Hemorrhoids can change the shape or texture of the anal opening. The perineum itself, the skin between the vagina and anus, may be longer or shorter or have a different texture.

It's disconcerting and not something most women have considered before having a baby.

Not all of the changes are permanent. Many scars will heal and become less visible, especially with proper scar care. Swelling will go down as bleeding lessens. Hemorrhoids can heal and go away. Yet some changes will remain, which can take time to grow into and adapt to. Our deep feelings about looking different are real. Our connection and attachment to our genital identity is real. These are not just any body parts. These are our sacred body parts, the ones through which we derive intimacy, unearth desires, and from which we created life. The exercises below can help you honor those feelings as well as grow into and evolve with any changes.

LOOKING IN THE MIRROR

One of the first ways to come home to yourself and your sexuality is to look at your vulva and vagina in a mirror. Check out how you look now. Take your time to look and notice the shape, the size, and the colors that you see. Notice the dimensions of your inner labia, your outer labia, and your perineum. Is the introitus, your vaginal opening, visible? As you look with your eyes, notice the sensations that arise in your body. As much as possible, maintain an attitude of curiosity. It is normal to feel strange if the look of your genitals has changed, and it probably has. Know that they probably will continue to change as your hormones shift, organs return to their place, ligaments get firmer, and healing continues.

You may want to do this a couple of times before your first postpartum visit so you witness your own progress. It can be fascinating to see all of the changes that your vulva goes through during the healing process. Many women worry that the changes to their genitals will be permanent and that sex will never be the same. While both may be true, women can gain full access to pleasure and sexual power, even with genitals that are different and new or changed desires with regard to sex.

VULVA BREATHING

....

Before reengaging with a partner and attempting to communicate your needs and desires, it is helpful to start by touching yourself. This doesn't have to be a self-pleasuring session, although it can be. Start by cupping your whole vulva with your hand. Send your breath all the way down through your belly and your pelvis, and feel your vulva expand into your hand. Imagine your mind is a flashlight illuminating parts of your body as your breath reaches them. You can follow your breath in through your nose and mouth, all the way through your throat, your heart, your deep belly, your pelvic bowl, and then contacting your hand. If there are gaps in that trail, just notice that. On the next breath, direct your mind and attention to the border zone of where you feel connected along this trail and where you don't. Linger at that border zone where your awareness gets murky, and notice if something changes. If it does, you may be able to feel farther along that trail. If not, continue to breathe and notice. This is a simple exercise connecting your breath and your attention to your vulva, and to softly and lovingly get in touch with her.

Your body went through a lot giving birth! You will have your own journey to meeting your intimate parts again. If the previous exercises feel like too much, vaginal steaming (chapter 6) is a gentle way to approach your vulva after giving birth. The steam actually feels good, so if you have an association with pain or discomfort or if you are averse to touching yourself, the steam can be a gentle buffer with the added benefits of cleansing your uterus and toning the tissues.

You should, of course, take your time with this, and proceed at your own comfort level. At the same time, just like a first bowel movement can feel scary, it's normal to feel some resistance to looking and feeling these intimate parts of yourself that may feel very different than they did before. Know that your feelings about your anatomy might not match what you see. I work with many women who are sure there is something wrong, misshapen, or out of place and when we explore together, they are pleasantly surprised that things are in place. Some women aren't quite sure what they looked like before, so don't have much to compare to. I also work with women who feel that things are very different, and they are. The texture, shape, and even what is visible externally can change after giving birth. Sometimes those changes are physically uncomfortable, sometimes they are emotionally disconcerting. In both cases, it's shocking. No one told us that our vulvas might be reshaped during birth.

If you avoid your vulva and vagina and your first attempt at penetrative sex is your reintroduction to this sensitive territory, you are setting yourself up for feelings of grief and confusion. Knowing our own anatomy, how it feels, how things work, and what we like are the first steps to being able to communicate what we want and feel when we decide to reengage sexually with a partner. After birth, partners will be looking for and needing your guidance about how to approach you again in a way that doesn't hurt and feels good for both of you. If you get to know what's happening with your vulva and vagina, so that penetrative sex is not your first reintroduction to this sensitive territory, you will be able to direct your sexual experiences, orienting toward pleasure.

SUMMARY

- To ensure full physical recovery—and not cause new symptoms—and to encourage pelvic-floor tone for your life, wait for six months before returning to running or heavy weight lifting.
- Specific pelvic-floor and core movements, called *bandhas*, are crucial in restoring inner health so that your return to exercise is successful.
- Your sexuality is your own. Begin by exploring your own body before returning to penetrative sex with your partner.

Reflections

- What does the phrase "your sexuality is your own" elicit in you?
- What is your experience of your body right now?

Exercises

- Practice the pelvic-floor visualizations and movements.
- Do a vaginal steam.
- Look at your vulva in a mirror, and practice vulva breathing.

reclaiming your sexuality

The postpartum time is a chance to create an even deeper and more satisfying sexual connection to ourselves and our partners, but things may not look like they looked before. In a culture where "maternal" and "sexual" are often seen as opposites, it's a radical act as a woman to refuse to succumb to this division within ourselves. Many women describe that they feel like virgins when they return to sex after having a baby, physically and emotionally. In many ways, this is 100 percent accurate. A new woman has been born. And this woman—this new mother—lives in a totally new body that has been reshaped and continues to change in innumerable ways. You are a new woman with a new body to explore and discover. This new woman, with her new and changing body, may have different needs and desires than the one who was left behind before pregnancy—and the one left behind before the baby exited.

Sexuality is about so much more than just sex. Sexuality activates our unconscious minds and can take us into liminal spaces, making it an extraordinary space for self-discovery, healing, and embodied learning. Sexuality has the potential to be the most transformative territory of our life. The postpartum time demands the redefinition and feminization of sex. Rather than sex being one more demand that drains us, sex can be an offering that fuels us. Rather than falling into a pattern of martyrdom, we can practice identifying our desires, asking for what we need, and placing our pleasure at the center. From that place, our erotic life can give us the energy we need to be present and to mother.

UNVEILING OUR ARCHETYPAL INHERITANCE

The way that we define ourselves and construct our identity is related to what is available in our cultural expressions of womanhood. The archetypes offered to us as women in the West are pretty limited—the maiden, mother, whore, and crone. Whether or not we are Christian, the Virgin Mary is the prevailing mother archetype. Her identity is based on separating her motherhood—which is combined with her spirituality—from sexuality. She was able to remain a virgin and become a mother. The only Western archetype that includes sexuality is the whore. So the Virgin Mother doesn't have sex to become a mother. The woman who does have sex is hidden and shamed. This is an expression of a belief not only that spirituality and sexuality are separate, but also that spirituality is good and higher and that sexuality is bad. Spiritual is pure and sexual is impure. Spiritual is clean and sexual is dirty. The Virgin Mary shows us that motherhood and sexuality don't go together. This dichotomy can consciously or unconsciously influence our sexuality during our motherhood journey.

Of course, there are many other archetypes and Goddesses around the world. Perhaps you grew up in a culture with totally different archetypes than those mentioned above. I have found a lot of comfort and inspiration in exploring the myth of Inanna, the Hindu Goddesses, representations of the Dark Feminine, and the Afro-Brazilian Goddesses. The exploration of how we create our own sexual identity from archetypes to family inheritance to personal experiences is so formative in how we experience the world that I created an online course to go deeper into just that, ultimately giving women more access to full sexual expression. You can find it here: www.vivainstitute.com/course/forging-a-feminine-path.

SEXUAL MOTHER

....

Explore your own ideas about motherhood and sexuality. Fold a piece of paper in half. At the top of one side, write "mother." On the top of the other side, write "sexual." Then list all the words you associate with "mother," and on the other side all the words you associate with "sexual." Do it quickly so you can capture your initial reactions. Then open the paper and look over your lists. Does anything surprise you?

FEMINIZING SEX

The postpartum time calls for the feminization of sex, which means placing a woman's pleasure at the center of each encounter. The majority of what we see and know about sex in our culture reflects male desires and male arousal. Pornography is a clear example of this. The orgasms that women have in porn are hard and fast, getting louder and louder as they escalate to a final peak and explosion. That trajectory reflects how many men experience arousal and climax. That version of climax has also influenced us as women with regard to what our pleasure should look like and sound like. We look for our experiences to match those images, whether unconsciously or consciously.

To place a woman's pleasure at the center, it's important to understand a few things about women's anatomy and women's arousal. Don't worry if this is new to you. It's new to almost everyone, for a whole bunch of reasons, including the fact that description of complete female sexual anatomy wasn't even included in anatomy books until recently.

Here are a few useful facts: The average time it takes for men to get aroused is thirty seconds to one minute. The average arousal time for most women is thirty-five to forty-five minutes. Sexual arousal is defined by the engorgement of the erectile tissue. Men and women have the same amount of erectile tissue, tissue that fills with blood and swells during arousal. In men, you can see the engorgement because their erectile tissue is mostly external and their penis changes shape and gets erect. Women also get "erect." Our vulvas get engorged and change shape, puffing up and flowering outward, but it takes much longer than it does for men. This is why "foreplay" is always suggested. I don't like the word *foreplay* because it suggests that something comes after and that you are working up to the main event, typically penetration. The feminization of sex means that we decondition ourselves to view sex as an act with a goal of penetration that ends in climax. Although there is nothing wrong with that, it narrows our experiences, our access to new potential pleasure pathways, and satisfaction with other ways of connecting. Everything that is considered "foreplay" is luscious and worthy of enjoyment for its own sake.

Many women have never experienced full arousal because of how much time it takes, and so have become accustomed to penetration before being fully aroused. Sheri Winston, the author of *Women's Anatomy of Arousal*, says that ideally penetration only happens when a woman is fully lubricated, totally aroused, and begging for it. While this may be new to you, that doesn't mean that sex hasn't been pleasurable for you. What it does mean is that there is a whole new world of pleasure awaiting!

After giving birth, our bodies are less forgiving when it comes to penetration without full arousal. I like to think of this as nature's way of nudging us toward deeper sexual exploration and creative connection.

Libido and True Desires

The fact is that few women want hard and fast penetration after having a baby. So they are tentative about sex because they don't know what to ask for or how to communicate it. Even when postpartum women say they have low libido, they are often open to sex and even want it; they just don't want the sex they are being offered. They want intimate connection that is relevant to them at that moment, not some old replay of how they did it before.

As women, most of us have been conditioned to believe that sex is something that we are giving, and that it is our job to please our partner. As new mothers we are already giving a good deal of energy, so it is a time to flip that script and allow our partners to please us. Most women don't want to receive affection when they know their partner is giving it only in hopes of getting more or going further, meaning any physical affection can start to feel like a demand. So it is time to flip the script that we owe our partner sex, and also that sex has to lead somewhere. As women, we are also taught that sex is a precious gift that we are giving away. We need to challenge that idea and identify what sex, in its broadest sense, can give us, and go after that.

JOURNALING YOUR DESIRES

Imagine if sex could be the very thing that gives you the energy you lack. Imagine if sex could recharge you, giving you energy instead of taking it from you.

- What kind of sex would that be?
- What would be one step closer to that kind of sex?

Take a moment to pull out your journal and a pen and brainstorm about this. Oftentimes, we are in touch with everything we don't want. Challenge yourself to think about what you do want. Ask yourself:

- What stands in my way of receiving?
- What stands in the way of asking for exactly what I want?
- What kind of touch do I absolutely love?
- What kind of touch am I curious about right now?
- What is an edge of resistance for me sexually but one that I am willing to explore?

This is an amazing opportunity to explore all the ways to be sensual, intimate, connected, and sexual without a destination. You might remember "Sex without Sex" from chapter 4. What can sex be like when penetration and even climax are off the table? What other ways can you connect that make you feel like you are in a sexual space together? What if just touching or kissing was just that—physical intimacy that didn't have the obligation of going further?

As foreign as your body and sexual identity may feel, your partner is waiting for your invitation and instructions. Lead him by asking for what you want, rather than avoiding or rejecting what you don't want. As noted above, our heterosexual culture defines sex as PIV penetration. While that may have been your definition and main way of connecting before baby, now is the time to expand your definition and experience of pleasure. Postpartum encounters should be guided by your pace of connection and your arousal levels.

If you haven't had a lot of open dialogue about your sexual relationship previously, the postpartum time, when everything feels so vulnerable, is not always the easiest time to start. Yet there is no other way than embracing radical honesty about how you are feeling, what you want, and then creating opportunities to engage and nurture that honesty and your intimacy. The communication exercises in chapter 10, "Deepening Intimacy," are a great place to start. Now it's time to include touch, to practice asking for what you want, and to practice checking in about what you have to give.

THE THREE-MINUTE GAME

I learned this game from Betty Martin, a revolutionary sex educator. There is so much to learn and explore in this very simple framework.

Begin with as broad of a definition of sex as possible, one that includes your whole body, mind, and spirit as an erogenous zone. Include sensuality, pleasure, and fantasy in your imagination. For our purposes right now, this game has two roles—giver and receiver. The giver's job is to give what is asked for and be receptive to any feedback from the receiver that would make his or her experience better. The job of the person giving is to be fully involved in giving, not just going through motions or wondering what it's going to lead to. The receiver's job is to ask for something that he or she truly wants to receive, and then communicate about what feels good and what could make it even better while receiving.

Now it's time to play the Three-Minute Game. Ask your partner for something you would like to receive. For example, "Would you play with my hair?" If he or she agrees to play with your hair, set a timer for three minutes. If your partner does not want to give what you asked for, he will suggest something else that he would like to give. Then, it is up to you to decide if you would genuinely like to receive that. If you don't want to, suggest something else, and continue until you find something that is a "yes" for both of you. This negotiation is an important part of the game: looking for the sweet spot of an option that is appealing to both people. This sets a precedent that both of your needs can be met. One of you doesn't have to lose while the other wins and gets what he or she wants. This might take creativity and some trial and error, but it's worth it.

Example:

R: Would you play with my hair?

G: (Pause to consider if you would like to) Yes.

Set the timer for three minutes.

R: I like the pressure you are using. Can you comb your four fingers from my hairline backward?

G: Yes. How's that?

R: That's perfect. Now can you grab a handful of hair and pull?

G: Yes. How's that?

R: Great.

G: Is there anything that would make it even more wonderful?

R: No, that's exactly what I want.

Example:

R: Will you passionately French kiss me?

G: No, but I'd like to feather kiss you all over your face.

R: (Pause to consider if he would like that) Yes, I would like that.

Set timer.

G: (lightly kissing) Is there anything that could make this more enjoyable?

R: Yes, if you linger a little longer before you make contact with my face, tease me a bit.

G: Thank you. (After a few moments) How's that? Shall I linger longer?

R: That's just right. Your timing is great.

Questions for the giver to ask the receiver:

Would you like more pressure?

Would you like a lighter touch?

Is there anything that could make this feel even better?

Givers can ask open-ended questions or questions about if the other person wants more or less of something. Receivers need to be specific with requests and direction.

When the three minutes are finished, allow for thirty seconds or so of silence and notice the sensations in your body. Then verbally share a moment that stood out for you. Decide together if you would like to play another round.

Here's a list of words describing ways to touch: tug, scratch, squeeze, tap, bite, lick, blow, rub, graze, brush, and knead. There are many more, but this is a good start. Have fun with it and request something you might not have experienced before.

Take the best parts of the Three-Minute Game and apply them to the rest of your intimate life. For example, if you are interested in kissing or another kind of intimacy but are wary of the expectations of what comes next, make clear requests. For instance, *I want to kiss for ten minutes without feeling like it has to go anywhere.* The time boundary can be comforting—a clear request with a clear time frame. Then, you can always choose to extend the timing.

I want to make sure everyone reading this book has as many tools as possible that will help them maintain their connection through their postpartum period. One tool that has been highly valuable for me, especially as a single mom who has been unpartnered for most of my journey and also had some sexual boundaries to repair is Orgasmic Meditation (OM). As a couple, this practice can take the pressure off of penetrative sex and offer a totally different way to connect. It's radical because it changes up ideas about giving and receiving, it places female pleasure at the center, and it takes climax off the table—many of the qualities of sexual interactions that are explored throughout this book.

OMing, as it is nicknamed, provides a fifteen-minute way to connect, where all that is asked of the woman is that she receive. The philosophy behind this practice is establishing clear boundaries and placing female pleasure, specifically the clitoris, at the center of the meditation. There is no pressure or goal of climax, just the goal of staying present with whatever arises as it arises. You can learn more about this practice and find a teacher near you at www.onetaste.us.

While penetrative sex is not the whole picture, eventually you will probably want to include it in your repertoire of sexual exploration and connection. There are some things you should know so that you can return to penetration in the most graceful and comfortable way possible.

After giving birth, our bodies are less forgiving when it comes to penetration without full arousal. There can be physical obstacles as well as psychological and mental ones that make it more difficult to engage when our bodies are not ready. Any kind of birth injury may create tenderness, both emotionally and physically. Our ability to lubricate can be affected by factors from hormones to breastfeeding to scar tissue. If our estrogen levels are low, the vaginal skin can feel thin and sensitive. Breastfeeding requires a lot of output of fluids, and your body may not be producing enough fluids for breast milk and vaginal lubrication. Scar tissue can block lubrication-producing glands. The ability to release fluids is also governed by the parasympathetic nervous system, so if you are feeling anxious or unable to relax, your body may not lubricate easily. To encourage lubrication, drink plenty of fluids and also don't be shy about using lube. And just as important, make sure that you are aroused and totally ready, mentally and physically, for penetration. Remember that each woman's timeline for this is different. There is no right timing for this. There is only your timing.

UNDERSTANDING THE LANDSCAPE

There are so many factors that contribute to how we experience sex postpartum and many of them are interrelated. Sex becomes like a tangled ball of yarn, the strands of pleasure, pain, intimacy, trauma, safety, and instinct are merged and interwoven. Differentiating what is playing into our desire or lack of it is not always straightforward. Many women feel a general sense of discomfort in their pelvis and vulva, feeling like things just "aren't right down there." As such, engaging sexually feels confusing and strange. Many women experience symptoms, like leaking urine when they sneeze, which again makes them feel like everything isn't right. So while they may or may not be afraid they might pee during sex, there is an overall distrust of how their sexual parts are functioning. They can't trust their body to feel and behave like it used to. The good news is when we parse out the strands from the tangled ball of yarn that usually gets labeled "low libido" or "I'm touched out," there are ways to address each of the strands.

If you feel ready but apprehensive about sex, the following is a list of some guidelines to keep in mind and possibly share with your partner.

....

"I was not prepared for how easily I could go into resentment—
my husband pulled his full share of parenting and house-holding,
but his household standards were lower and different than mine,
and this was exacerbated when I felt I didn't have it in me to
tend to the house but couldn't stand the state it was in. I lost
perspective on how messy or not it actually was in any abso-
lute sense. I could get mad at my husband on a dime, and
his acceptance of me didn't help. I would get pissed if he got
sleep, pissed if he stayed up playing bass or doing something
else objectively enjoyable or frivolous. The amount of loving
attention you need to give to a primary relationship is huge,
because if attended to, that relationship nourishes your parenting, your sense of self, your sense of peace in your life.

"Even though I didn't deliver vaginally in the end, my vagina,
cervix, and uterus were entirely rearranged. It felt like playing
pin the tail on the donkey while drunk to have sex—all angles
felt wrong, there was no sweet spot. This was for a good long
while and only changed once we found some exquisite lube and,
of course, over time with the natural return to alignment. It was
really unfortunate because sex is a big source of connection
between my husband and me—it doesn't replace other forms
of love and intimacy, but for him this was a big loss and for me
it sucked that I felt so raw and tender down there. Then once
things healed I would sometimes have to choose between
sleep and sex. Though sleep always seemed more urgent, I can
tell you that actually sometimes the closeness and physical
relaxation that came from sex was more important."

For Comfortable, Connected Sex Postpartum

- Clear away resentments.
- Let your partner know that you desire them; share appreciations.
- Connect daily for one to five minutes through eye gazing or gentle touch.
- Enjoy the journey and forget about the destination.
- Use lubrication liberally if you need it.
- Communicate desires in the present moment.
- Allow the woman's pleasure to be the guide of the encounters.
- Ask for what you want, even if you are not sure you will get it.
- Approach each other anew each day.
- Allow sensual, connected, and intimate to be in the "sexual" category too.
- After the fourth trimester, schedule time once a week for two to three hours of open-ended connection.

As mentioned above, you may experience some discomfort or apprehension the first few times that you return to penetrative sex. However, sex should never be painful. If it is painful, there is a reason for it. Once you know what may be contributing to the pain, seek support to address it so that you can feel that you have full access to your body and you are comfortable again. Everything in the list below has been mentioned in other chapters of the book, but use this list to troubleshoot and ask yourself honestly if any of these symptoms are part of what is contributing to your willingness to approach sex right now.

What May Contribute to Difficult or Painful Penetration

- Birth injury
- Sensitive tissue
- Scar tissue
- Dehydration

- Unfinished birth energy
- Birth trauma
- Lack of mental or emotional readiness
- Resentments
- Insufficient arousal (not enough time spent in pleasure before penetration)
- Previous trauma in the area

All of the above scenarios and feeling-states are possible contributors to why sex may be difficult to approach and they have been addressed in earlier chapters. If you have a birth injury of any kind, scar tissue from tearing or stitching, sensitive tissue, prolapse, or incontinence, seek help from a holistic pelvic health-care specialist, pelvic floor physical therapist, or STREAM trained practitioner. If you have birth trauma or unfinished birth energy beyond what you were able to address through the exercises in this book, seek out Somatic Experiencing trauma resolution therapy, Hakomi therapy, visionary cranio-sacral work, some other body-based healing modality, or the Birth Story Medicine work of Pam England.

If you don't feel ready or have resentments or unresolved relationship dynamics, communicate bravely or seek couples' counseling for support in communicating. If there is insufficient arousal, take more time in transition into sexual space before genital touch, so that penetration sounds appealing. If there isn't enough lubrication, make sure you are drinking enough fluids. If you have given yourself ample time for arousal before penetration (at least thirty minutes), use a lubricant to decrease friction on sensitive tissues. Lubrication will also increase when you stop breastfeeding. If your birth scenario has activated previous trauma, seek out a guide whether a counselor, mentor, therapist, or shaman to help shepherd you through the process of integrating these earlier experiences into your new identity.

Community Stories:
Brenda

A few sessions into our work together, Brenda confided to me that becoming a mother was really changing her relationship to her body and her sexuality. She shared that she had always felt that spirituality was the most important thing in her life. Although she had distanced herself from rigid religious beliefs, she was someone whose faith was palpable. When she said "God," what she meant was *love*—the love that is home for everyone. But she had always seen the spiritual as opposite to the sexual. Because she wanted to be a spiritual person, she didn't want to see herself as a sexual person.

When we talked about desires, her main want was not to shut her husband down in exploring his desires. It was hard for her to identify any desires of her own. In our sessions together, she returned each time brighter and brighter. Just identifying how she had seen spiritual and sexual as opposites set in motion a process of self-acceptance and loving-kindness, as she described it. She gave herself permission to be fully present with sex itself. When I mentioned the idea of maintenance sex, when women are counseled to have sex even when they don't want it to keep their partners happy, she said, "Yes! That's what I was doing 70 percent of the time *before* I had a baby." She mentioned that having a daughter had also set off this cascade of inquiry for her: How did she want to talk about sexuality to her daughter? How did she want to embody sexuality as a model for her daughter?

The sexual life that she was enjoying with her husband felt less separate from the rest of her life now. She didn't feel like she had "jump over a fence to the sexual side" as she put it.

There wasn't regular Brenda and Brenda who had to gear up to have sex; they were one and the same. She also stated that accepting her sexual self was a part of self-love for her. Brenda was beautifully maturing into her sovereign sexual identity together with her mother identity, as she decided to be fully present and allow herself to enjoy her intimate sexual life with her husband. She was also learning about the continuity of connection that can include our sexual experience.

We don't have to acquiesce to the message that our sex lives are over, nor do we have to force ourselves into an image of what good lovers or wives "should do." We need to get quiet and listen to the whispers of our desires. We need to honestly communicate what we want, which changes each moment of each day. With our new bodies and new identities, we need to courageously face our new partner, creating an even tighter bond from which the family can grow. We embrace a feminine identity that doesn't have to be expressed in only one way. We don't have to choose between being spiritual and being sexual. We don't have to choose between being a mother and being sexual. We can be spiritual and sexual. We can be a mother and be sexual.

We are forging a new path of womanhood that can include motherhood, sexuality, and spirituality so that the next generation can enjoy equal rights without giving up feminine embodiment.

SUMMARY

- The Virgin Mary represents a separation between motherhood and sexuality. Integrating our mother selves and sexual selves is a radical act.
- Reclaiming sex includes redefining sex and feminizing sex.

- Most women feel as if they are starting over again with their sexual identity and desires after having a baby. This can be an invitation into a more authentic sexual expression.
- Sex should never be painful. If it is, there is a reason for it. Assess what you think the source of pain is so that you can get the right support.

Reflections

- What are some of the sexual scripts that you recognize as a part of your belief system?
- What kind of touch do you absolutely love?
- What kind of touch are you curious about right now?
- What is the relationship between sexuality and spirituality in your life? Are they interconnected ideas or totally separate?

Exercises

- Fold a piece of paper in half. At the top of one side, write "mother." On the top of the other side, write "sexual." Then list all the words you associate with "mother," and on the other side all the words you associate with "sexual." Do it quickly so that you can capture your initial reactions. What surprises you?
- Play the Three-Minute Game as both giver and receiver. Another day, play the Three-Minute Game in the receiving role only.
- Take the next step in engaging your sexuality by learning the Orgasmic Meditation practice at onetaste.us or join Forging a Feminine Path at www.vivainstitute.com/course/forging-a-feminine-path/.

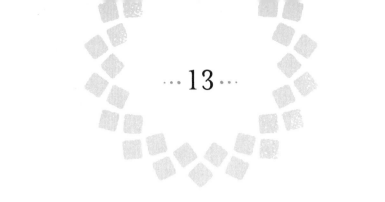

··· 13 ···

discovering the mother you are

The best thing we can teach any mother is how to listen to her intuition, how to go inside and find her inner voice. The greatest pediatricians, educators, and psychologists, from Dr. Sears to Maria Montessori to Laura Gutman, have all contended that it is mothers that truly know the needs of their children. They have suggested that professionals should sharpen their listening skills to hear what mothers already know about their babies. The problem is that with the sheer amount of information available through the Internet, new mothers are more swamped than ever with opinions about how to do things and what is best for their babies.

When we become mothers, the voices of our own grandmothers and mothers awaken within us. Visceral memories, whether explicitly recalled or implicitly felt, surface. Cultural messages abound. We are inundated by cultural, familial, and personal scripts about what the right way to raise a child is. At a vulnerable time, when our hormones are in flux and our identity is forming and re-forming, we are not always clear about who's leading the way with our decision-making. Our thoughts and ideals may change when confronted with having to make actual decisions with our real baby in front of us. We may shift our priorities in ways we wouldn't have expected. We are pushed to mature, bridging the gap between our ideals, our capacities, real-world considerations, and the individual needs of the baby we birth.

FINDING YOUR STYLE OF MOTHERING

From crying it out to co-sleeping, there is no shortage of professional and personal opinions about the best way to raise a child. The pressure to find the best parenting style is intense. Some of these choices seem so critical to assuring our babies' long-term health—and our chances of getting a decent night's sleep—that women can feel paralyzed with indecision. We are deeply influenced by what we do or don't want to repeat about our own childhoods, and we also can't help but keep an eye on what is happening with our friends and the families around us. Worse yet is the influence of social media, showing us a stilted view of what other families are like, where we consistently see only the highlights. How do we find our own voices in the midst of so much input and feedback?

BODY COMPASS

Here's one way to get in touch with your intuition or felt sense that can be a reliable compass for decision-making. Remember that intuition and rational thought are different skills. Intuition is a heart and body experience. Rational thought is a head experience. Intuition doesn't require reasons or explanations. It is just a gut feeling, something you simply know. Right now, we are practicing sensing in the body. You can do this with eyes closed or open. Feeling internal sensations is often easier with eyes closed.

- Settle in to a comfortable posture—lying down, sitting, or standing. Close your eyes so that you can feel your internal sensations more clearly. (If you prefer, you can also keep your eyes open, softly focused on a point out in front of you.)
- When you have a question about something like, "Should I go pick up my baby or let her cry longer?" or "Is now the right time to introduce food?" call that question to mind. Choose just one question and be specific, such as: "Should I go pick up my baby right now?"

- Notice what sensations arise in your body. You may notice story lines appear, such as, "What kind of mom are you to let your baby cry?" or "You are such a pushover that you keep going to get her." See if you can notice these as story lines, and not the whole picture. It may help to label them as story or thought.
- You may notice emotions arise—confusion or guilt or feeling overwhelmed. Notice these, and label them too.
- Then, see if you can turn your attention to your body sensations. Somewhere in your body, there is a "gut feeling." Maybe it is actually in your gut. Some women feel intuition in their womb. Discover the place in your body where intuition lives for you.
- Place your hand on this spot. Ignoring the circling thoughts and emotions, ask your specific, clear, and yes-or-no question again, and listen for the answer from this place.

At first, it is best to practice this while being still, but after you practice, you can do this anytime, anywhere. Just check in with your body and see what answer your body gives you. Have fun experimenting with simple choices like which route to take to the grocery store or what you feel like for dinner. It will then become easier with more difficult choices.

Every mother will be faced with difficult choices, but when we are true to ourselves and what we know is right for ourselves and our babies, we gain strength in our decision-making.

After my daughter was born, I couldn't walk for a few months due to the birth injury, so it made sense for us to sleep in the same bed. I was able to nurse well lying down, so I got good sleep that way, and I had planned to co-sleep for the first six months anyway. Over the first three years of my daughter's life, my parents bought two cribs in hopes that my daughter would sleep in one. My mom bought the first one in Brazil, before my daughter was born. To my mom, baby equaled crib. I didn't like the idea of cribs, with the bars in the baby's visual awareness.

Community Stories:
Agatha

....

Agatha called me on a Friday afternoon, at the end of the first week that her husband had gone back to work after their twins were born. They had just come from the pediatric dentist, who had told her that both children were tongue-tied and lip-tied. Tongue-ties are when the frenulum, the thin piece of skin that attaches the tongue to the bottom of the mouth, is short so that the baby cannot move its tongue well enough for nursing. A lip tie is when the frenulum that connects the lip to the gums is too short, also complicating nursing. Prior to going, she thought maybe her son was having difficulty, but she had no idea that her daughter, who seemed to be nursing incredibly well, would also receive this diagnosis.

On the verge of tears, she lamented that she had no idea what to do.

I asked her to pause for a moment and notice her breath. I reminded her that it was Friday afternoon after a long week, both babies were doing really well, and there was no emergency. I asked if she had had enough to eat in the last few hours. She told me everything she had done that day, and I knew she was exhausted. I told her to put any decision-making on hold until the following day, during the weekend, when she and her husband could discuss the options together. I reminded her that they both had great instincts, and I knew that they would be able to feel what was right for them. Because a new mother's biological directive is to protect her children, the brain is wired to worry as a mechanism of protection. We have to remind ourselves to distinguish between real crises and what our systems perceive as crises because we are tired, overwhelmed, and primed to look for what is wrong.

The following week Agatha returned to her lactation consultant and discovered that her babies weren't getting as much food as they needed. Again, she called me in tears, overwhelmed by all the options and opinions. Clip their tongues? Feed them formula? Pump all the time? She was considering supplementing one feeding a day with formula. But she was still worried about the lip-tie-tongue-tie situation and worried she would mess up her milk supply with bottle-feeding. The thought of pumping every feeding in addition to breastfeeding twins was pushing her over the edge.

I asked her, "Agatha, what does your gut say? What is your gut telling you to do?"

Without missing a beat, she said, "My gut is telling me to give them one bottle a day."

"Do that then. The idea of pumping a lot sounds like it's very stressful for you. What if you just pumped when you had the energy to? What if you didn't force yourself into it? I am concerned that if you push yourself too hard here, you might enter into a counterproductive pattern. Making enough breast milk hinges on you being relaxed. You are feeding two human beings and healing from an abdominal surgery. You need to choose the option where you are not sacrificing yourself. What is the option that is best for the four of you? What is the option that includes your sanity and well-being? That day she began supplementing.

We need to remind mothers that underneath everyone else's opinions, medical advice, and even their own conflicting internal voices, they can contact their intuition. Mothers almost always know what is best for their babies.

To my mom's credit, she also bought me a baby dresser that doubled as a changing table, and it turned out to be very necessary!

When I came back to the United States, my mom bought another crib, in the hopes that I would establish a routine where my daughter would be able to stop co-sleeping. She eventually sold it when we moved back to Brazil. Neither of those cribs was ever used.

Over the years, many people suggested that co-sleeping was negatively affecting both my daughter and me. Some people suggested that I could never have a romantic relationship if she was occupying that space in my bed. A Freudian analyst suggested that if I had erotic dreams, they would unconsciously and inappropriately affect my daughter. My parents were so frustrated when my daughter stayed with them because she didn't have a normal bedtime routine. She needed to be sleeping next to one of them to fall asleep. This went on for years, and it felt like I was constantly receiving input that I was doing something potentially damaging. At times, I was swayed and thought it was ridiculous that she was five and still sleeping with me. I was a slave to this nighttime routine, always having to put her to bed. So I would mount a campaign, buy new, frilly bedsheets, and make a big deal out of this symbolic step of her growing up. Typically she would get in her new bed, we'd read a book, kiss good night, I'd walk over to my bed and lie down, and after about five minutes of silence, she'd walk over to my bed and ask "Can I just get in?" and I would concede. The truth was that we both loved it—until we didn't.

While I was writing chapter 9, on birth stories, I had a realization about why my daughter and I were still sleeping together in the same bed. As I wrote about how birth stories have powerful information and keys to our souls' journeys and our relationships with the people who were present at the birth, I decided that it was time for me to take my own advice.

When I was left alone for a few hours during the transition time of her labor, we had embedded an internal conviction that it was the two of us against the world. That thought had remained with us.

As long as we continued to return to this most primary bond every night, my daughter would always insist that we sleep in one of two physical positions, reminiscent of the positions she nursed in, and would be distraught if I wanted to change things.

I needed to show her in a visceral and somatic way that she and I would be okay without sleeping together each night. I wanted her to feel that there are other reliable pillars of support in life other than me. The idea of it startled her a bit. I gave her a week's notice and assured her that she could still cuddle in the morning. This time, the plan actually worked! It had never worked when I was trying to get her out of my bed because other people were telling me that I should. Changing the habit worked when I was truly ready. When, deep in my bones, I felt it was what was right, I was able to withstand the opposition she was going to mount.

I feel it is also important to mention that I had several great relationships during this time. The chorus of opinions chiming in from outside that suggested that I was sabotaging my ability to have romantic relationships and was making a grave error did not prove true, at least not in the ways that people insinuated.

As you go through this tenderizing process that is parenting, you will also realize that it is less about getting it right and more about figuring out who you are, who your child is, and who you are together. Was co-sleeping the right decision? I can't say. Would I do it again? I don't know. But I do know that co-sleeping was part of our unique dance together that was ours to live. I know that changing this pattern had its own timing and required deep inquiry, attunement, and courage. I believe that the separation happened when we were both ready for it and could sustain the change.

This is no treatise for or against the idea of co-sleeping. This is simply to illustrate that every single choice we make has pros and cons. Any parenting model can be tyrannical if we don't allow ourselves to live and breathe inside of it. We are constantly weighing our needs against our babies' needs to make the choice that is best for both of us, because what we think is best for *them* may not be what is actually best for *us*. We are constantly forced to place our ideals on the cutting board. In fact, these ideologies or styles of parenting torture us when we feel we *must* follow them, because the experts or books know better than we do.

The truth is that no method will give us the key to unlock the mysteries of our babies. We cling to methods and styles when we feel out of control, and who doesn't as a new parent? We feel like if we just do the right thing and figure it out, our babies will stop crying or learn to sleep better or be a genius or whatever it is that we are trying to accomplish. Author and mother Leonie Dawson wrote on her blog, "Parenting is one hard bugger of a ride. So overwhelming and threatening that we think—if only I find the One Thing That Will Make It All Right, I will prescribe my life to it and not deviate from its plan. But the plan we are meant to be living is our own. The one that makes us all joyful, glad, happy and easy."

It's hard to feel emotionally stable when we're constantly questioning our own decisions and, more than that, when "helpful" friends, family members, and health professionals are questioning them as well. So it's important to remember and remind yourself often that just because one person—or even five—suggest something, that doesn't mean it's right for you. Consider anything else in your life: your relationships, your career path, even your decisions to cut your hair. Friends and family and experts will always suggest certain things they've seen work, but when it comes down to it, you will, most likely, take what they say, assess how you feel about the situation, and then make your decision based on that.

If you've tried the Body Compass exercise and are still having trouble getting in touch with your intuition about a decision, try journaling.

WRITING TO FIND YOUR INTUITION

....

List some of the suggestions that you've been told by people—to pump, not to pump, to co-sleep, not to co-sleep, to wean at six months, to nurse till two years—and then write down your initial responses without censoring or giving in to the voices that chime in about how you "should" feel or what you should do. Leave it for a day or two. Then, return and write down your more thought-out responses or other considerations that might not have come up right away. Also, make room for how you feel now, which might not be how you felt before you met this baby. Each baby is unique, and the mother you are may change with each baby. You also might notice that the voices of certain people factor very strongly in your decisions—either in agreeing with them or disagreeing with them. It's important to understand what is coming from your authentic values and what is coming from your social group or your family.

One of the most dominant inner voices will probably be your mother's or your grandmother's.

IDENTIFYING YOUR MOTHER LINEAGE

In becoming mothers, our experience of being mothered is reawakened. Our feelings about our first relationship—our relationship with our mothers—and the mother-daughter connection can come to the surface during this heightened time. Becoming mothers brings us into the experience of attaching to an infant, and in doing so, we may become aware of how we were able to attach, or not, to our own mothers as children. Women who were adopted may experience a feeling of disorientation or displacement that is reminiscent of their own infancy, when they were separated from their own kin and were delivered into a totally new environment to be raised. Not only are we raising babies, but we are also encountering ourselves at those ages as we meet our own babies at these ages. Because of this, our feelings toward our own mothers are often magnified.

During the first few months of my daughter's life, I was awestruck by what it actually takes to be a mother. I felt a profound sense of gratitude for both my mother and my father. They actually did this for me. They fed me. They rocked me. They stayed up all night with me. They changed my diapers. They were confounded by me. They lost sleep over me. My mom spent six weeks trying to nurse me while her mom told her it wasn't worth it and to just give up. My mom pushed me, a nine-and-a-half-pound baby, out of her body. She did that for me.

In my bones, I felt that there are very few mothers that don't deeply love their children. How well they love is another question entirely, but the presence of love is undeniable. I realized after I gave birth that having my own mother at the birth of my daughter would have made all the difference in my ability to relax. My mom would have noticed that the bath water was not warm enough, that I needed a rubber band to tie up my hair that I kept wrangling out of my face. She would have understood my words and my facial expressions. In the same way that I can often finish her sentences, my mom would have known what I needed.

After I gave birth, my mom was the only one I felt comfortable showing my stitches to, the only one who seemed to understand the gravity of what I was going through. It was my mom who confirmed for me that the tear was not healing normally. It was my mom to whom I could hand my daughter off and then sleep deeply, without an ounce of apprehension or doubt that she would be well taken care of. My mom and I have not always had a smooth relationship. I was a sassy, disrespectful teenager and have been apologizing ever since. As a young adult, I went through important but painful periods of time without speaking to her. We have had our share of ruptures and repairs. Perhaps that is why I was so surprised that, in spite of having defined myself in opposition to her for much of life, when I became a mother, I gained respect for her. Standing in the same role together, as mothers, I saw her differently.

I believe that if I had grown up in almost any other culture, I may have already had that respect. But as Americans, we are not only allowed to dislike our mothers, we can talk openly about it. We are permitted to reject our elders—not just their ways but the people themselves. However, after women become mothers, that narrative seems to change. Most women see their mothers in a different, more positive light. Giving birth gave me a welcome wake-up call. If the Buddhists say to treat every being as if they had once been your mother, consider: How do you treat your actual mother?

Community Stories:
Shirley

"I now know how she sees me. How, to her, despite all of our battles, my anger, her anger, my disconnectedness, her inability to remember the darkest times . . . despite all of this . . . I am a type of angel to her. She remembers how deeply she loved me when we first met. And, that love resides strongly in the core of her psyche. She is Mother. She has and will do anything for her children. I now understand this. Our relationship feels different now that I have also given birth. There is a type of shared female equivalence. She sees that I am now Mother . . . and less daughter. We speak to each other more as women . . . and less like relatives. I see that she sees the deep love I have for my child, I see that she sees my struggles. She sees that I see this, and she has softened toward me. She allows me to take the lead as Mother, but stands by in support, gently offering advice when she senses I could use some help. I have softened toward her . . . and become less self-centered in our relationship. I have moved toward meeting her in the middle, and she stands calmly, graciously . . . and accepts me. Also, our relationship has strengthened through a shared, sacred bond—her only grandchild, my only child."

As our identity shifts into *mother*, who we are in the role as a daughter changes. Many women find themselves straddling the fence of how they feel as a mother and how they feel as a child. No matter how resolved we think we may be with our relationship to our mothers, no matter how individuated or how over it we think we are, another layer arises when we give birth. It's a time when we need mothering, and if we don't receive it from either our own mothers or from someone who can serve as a surrogate mother, we are thrown back into reliving all of the ways that we didn't receive it in the past. We may feel a sense of helplessness, isolation, abandonment, or anger. We feel our present need to be mothered simultaneously with all of our younger selves who also needed to be mothered. There is legitimate and palpable grief. It is not hard to see how women who are grieving their mother relationship together with a traumatic birth or birth injuries are likely to have a more difficult time recovering from birth.

Community Stories:
Maggie

I thought I would only be a mother after I had a child. I didn't realize I would also continue to still be a child. I was seeing my own mother through my new bifocals: me as a child judging her actions, "Wow, you really fucked that up"; and me as a mother judging her actions, "My word, you shined in a storm." I had to call her the day I came to a part in the novel I was reading about a woman who with love, grace, and terror leaves her children to pursue another life. My own mother had left me for a bit when I was young. Now that I had a child I finally understood how a mother could do such a thing. I also sat with myself the child and still wondered: "How could you have done that to me?"

But there is another painful side to the story for women who were not mothered well. When there is unprocessed emotion, the postpartum period can become heavier and more intense. For women who have contentious and difficult relationships with their mothers, they can be ricocheted back into their childhood selves, left wondering if any of the work they did on themselves earlier made any impact at all. These women often suffer in confusion and silence, blaming themselves for not feeling the warm-and-fuzzy thoughts toward their own mothers that they hear other new moms espousing.

WRITING TO YOUR MOTHER

Whether your relationship to your mother is mostly heartening or mostly painful, give voice to your inner selves—you as daughter and you as mother. There may even be multiple voices of you as a daughter at different ages. Write your thoughts and feelings in the form of a letter to your mother. Tell her what you want her to know. You don't have to send it to her. Give yourself permission to say exactly what you think, exactly how you feel, without censoring yourself.

- Write your mother a letter from you as a mother.
- Write your mother a letter from you as a child.

After giving birth, we are called to expand and hold these seemingly conflicting and, at times, even warring perspectives. Although we may have compassion for how our mothers were themselves mothered and their particular challenges, the abandoned, hurt, and frantic child in us also needs a voice and needs space. At this time, we need to give ourselves a long leash of compassion for acting out, being short-tempered, unpredictable, and yes, maybe even immature.

In the midst of these maddening and competing pulls (and maybe even because of them) as well as what feels like overwhelming darkness, maturity is happening. We recognize that the process of mothering itself is helping us re-mother ourselves. We don't usually learn much about ourselves when everything is going exactly as planned. In this tumult, there is the chance to realize that there is nothing in us that is beyond repair—because deep inside, there is the truth of who we are that is enduring and strong.

Our relationships to our mothers affects everything including our physical health. Women's health pioneers such as Dr. Christiane Northrup and Maya Tiwari suggest that it is our relationship to our mother that sits at the headwaters of our health. When women come to them with any kind of health problem, but especially with gynecological or reproductive problems, they ask their patients to look honestly at their relationships to their mothers. The following exercise guides you through some basic inquiries about what you would like to carry forward in your lineage and what you would like to leave behind. It can be easy to focus on the negatives, so it is especially important to include the parts you would like to continue.

MOTHER LINEAGE TREE

Get a large piece of paper. Draw a circle in the center in the bottom third of the page. Put your name above the circle and then divide the circle in half with a vertical line. Diagonally to your circle, in the upper left, write your mother's name above another circle. Then place your grandmother's name above another circle on that high diagonal. Diagonally to the right and up from your circle, write your father's name above a circle, and then continue with his mother's name above a circle. Divide all the circles in half. On the left half of the circle, write out the positive qualities of the person that you liked or loved. On the right half of the circle, place the qualities of the person that you don't like, ones that may be negative or damaging. Then come down to your circle. On the left side, place the qualities from your mother's side that you want to pass on to your child. On the right side, list the qualities from your father's side that you want to carry on as part of your legacy.

So many unconscious family patterns get awakened when we become parents that it is important to be conscious about what we want to offer as our legacy. While we may be very clear about patterns we want to break, acknowledging our roots and what is deep in us that we have to offer our children is life affirming.

In so many ways, the postpartum period exposes the deficiency of the nuclear family model. We know it takes a village to raise a child. It also takes a village to raise a mother! Women need other women around during early mothering as reflections and reminders that everything is going to be okay. Women need permission to fall apart and to know that someone will keep things together as they reassemble themselves. Women need to be able to dive into the depths with other women who have also been in the depths, as reminders that there is a way out and another side. When we can not only see but also experience how many versions there are of being mothered and mothering, we have a broader palette to choose from in how we will mother. As we become more receptive to being mothered by different women, we also model for our children that we are not going to be and cannot be everything for them. We teach them to value trust and the depth of support that happens when you get it from many sources, and we stop making ourselves sick trying to single-handedly occupy myriad roles that are meant to be occupied by many.

We model trust in life that they and we will be taken care of, even if not from unexpected directions. We widen the net of interconnectedness.

NEGOTIATING SINGLE MOTHERHOOD

If finding a community or village or tribe is important for mothers in relationship, it is even more important for single mothers. Women become single mothers in all different ways. Some women are single mothers by choice and plan to be the sole providers for their child. Other women enter into parenting wanting or expecting it to be a joint endeavor with their partners but end up with sole responsibility. Still others may have experienced unexpected loss that led them to single motherhood.

The assumption most people have, including us single mothers at times, is that two parents, a mother and a father, are what is best for a child. Our position as single women who are mothers challenges this, and often people are relating to stereotypes of what it means to be a single mother rather than who we are as individuals. Movies show single mothers struggling to make ends meet, making bad choices in men, and down on their luck.

If locating ourselves within our archetypal inheritance of maidens, virgin mothers, and prostitutes is complex for partnered mothers, as explored in chapter 12, locating ourselves within these choices is additionally complicated for single mothers. We simply don't fit into the categories that are offered. Our existence creates questions for people. Figuring out how much of our personal life to disclose and to whom is a daily dilemma. Helping our children understand and navigate those questions is also an ongoing inquiry as they grow.

However women become single mothers, we end up in the position of occupying both the masculine and the feminine roles in parenting, which can feel like an oppressive amount of responsibility at times. There is less leeway for us to lose it, because there is no one to stay in the house while we go for a walk around the block.

While living in isolation is stressful for all mothers, it is especially taxing for single mothers. We need even more practical help and emotional support. The postpartum period is a time when all women need to be surrounded by other women; it can be devastating to be alone as a new mother. It can be very difficult to get out of the house with a new baby, but make sure that you do not go days on end without contact with other adults. As single mothers, we have to be resourceful in how we can get the nurturing and holding that we need. We have to creatively find ways to meet our erotic needs outside of partnership. We have to rally neighbors, friends, family, and our community and allow ourselves to receive all the help that is offered. If you are finding this book after already having given birth, refer to the Postpartum Sanctuary Plan now (chapter 3 and appendix 1), and assemble and deepen your resource pool. Finding a network of other single mothers is invaluable, not only to coordinate childcare, housekeeping, and food preparation, but also for solidarity in an experience that is hard for people to understand who haven't done it themselves.

Single mothers often feel guilt about their child only having one parent and about the limits of what one parent can provide. It's important to know that what every child needs is one parent who is attuned to him or her. So if you can put energy toward your own sanity and well-being, then you will have the patience and clarity you need to stay connected to your baby. Our babies don't require perfection, they require our attention. As the sole parent, you can also look forward to a very close bond with your child.

Becoming a Good Enough Mother

After working with thousands of mothers and children, English pediatrician and psychoanalyst D. W. Winnicott coined the phrase "good enough mother" to explain the notion that our fallibility as mothers will not necessarily traumatize our children. Oftentimes, the multitude of child-rearing opinions, styles, and methods is overwhelming, but more paralyzing is that we all imagine our children will be permanently damaged by these choices. The good news is that Winnicott found that repair is always possible. He calls the mistakes we make "ruptures," some of which are absolutely necessary as a part of life. He calls the correction of a rupture a "repair," and he encourages mothers to make thoughtful repairs. Instead of avoiding ruptures, we do well to turn our attention to the repair that builds security in the relationship. With a good enough mother, the child knows that her relationship to her mother can withstand ruptures. She can count on the return of safety and love.

A good enough mother knows that imperfect circumstances are part of life. A good enough mother is a three-dimensional human being who is both selfless and selfish. A good enough mother is a real mother with real considerations, real concerns, and real flaws in the real world. A good enough mother protects space for herself to look inward at the same time she looks outward, toward the needs of her children and other loved ones. Good enough mothers are allowed not to love all aspects of mothering all the time—yes, that's right. We are not required to always love and enjoy parenting.

It's amazing how even the permission to not like some aspects of mothering can feel blasphemous. I wrote an article that expressed that I have a major deficit in the housekeeping department. If cleaning and cooking are genetic, I definitely inherited a double recessive. I talked about other parts of motherhood that I don't like. I was shocked that being a mom was like being a producer, and I am terrible at organization. I am continually surprised by how much of mothering is physical and logistical. In response to this part of my article, one mother commented, "I had no idea I was allowed to feel this way. I had no idea I was allowed to admit that there were parts of this process that I hate." Indeed, Winnicott said it was healthy for mothers to give themselves permission to hate it some of the time. I like to think that that permission is what allows us the space to genuinely love it some of the time.

What parts of mothering have surprised you? What do you genuinely dislike or even hate about mothering? What do you enjoy about mothering?

LEARNING TO NOT CHASE PERFECTION

When my daughter was six weeks old, my milk supply was very low. As a result, she was nursing all the time and was often irritated, as she was without enough nourishment. As I ingested everything from rice pudding to fennel tea to dark beer to try to build my milk supply, I worried that I was giving my daughter an eating disorder. I worried that maybe I was creating a lifelong pattern of desperation because she was suffering as I struggled to maintain my ideal of exclusively breastfeeding her until she reached six months old. To me it was unfathomable that a mother could not make enough milk for her own child. How could nature make such a highly impractical and un-Darwinian error? I could not see the tremendous pressure I was under recovering from the birth, living far away from my family and friend network, and buckling under an unstable relationship—so I resisted. I went to the milk bank every day, receiving different advice each time.

One day, when I was sitting in the park, my daughter was fussing and restlessly shifting from breast to breast and back again. By my side was a mother whose two-month-old baby was as big as a linebacker. He was satiated after nursing just half of one of her enormous breasts. When she saw what was going on with me, she offered to nurse my daughter. With a teary feeling of surrender and gratitude, I passed my baby over—something I never would have imagined myself doing. My daughter nursed nonstop for ten minutes and then fell fast asleep. In that moment, I realized that I had to give up my imagined ideal in favor of something that made sense for our situation. I began supplementing with breast milk from friends. When that ran out, I used formula, whose ingredients included hydrogenated vegetable oil because it was the only one available in Brazil at the time. At four months, my daughter cut teeth. I decided to drop the formula and introduce food, and my milk supply caught up. I had to make the best choice from what was available, which was one of the first of many compromises when reality prevailed over my ideals.

Recently, while learning from one of my teachers, the birth visionary Pam England, she asked a mother she was coaching how she would rate herself as a mother on a scale from 1 to 7. The woman gave herself a 5 or a 6. Pam applauded her and went on to explain that we don't want to be perfect mothers. If she had given herself a 7, her partner would probably have given her a 2—she also probably wouldn't be very happy with her own life, and moreover, her kids wouldn't develop the resilience they needed. Agreeing with Winnicott, Pam explained that not only do children not need perfect mothers, but that it's actually not good for children to have perfect mothers. Well, I had certainly never thought of it that way, but it made perfect sense to me. This was a huge revelation, and I felt like I'd received a cosmic permission slip when I heard it. What a relief! I was actually being in the service of my daughter by not being perfect.

Making mistakes, apologizing, and experimenting are all parts of being human. More and more, research shows that for growth and excellence, learning how to fail is much more important than succeeding on a first try. We want to teach and model failing and resilience to our children. Learning that it's okay to fail takes more than someone telling you it's okay and then demanding perfection of themselves. We all learn through modeling; kids learn through seeing adults make mistakes and then recovering and starting again. Children need to see their mothers' missteps and corrections. It is modeled permission—not verbal permission—they need in order to develop the ability to take risks and grow.

JOURNALING ON MOTHERHOOD, PERFECTIONISM, AND LETTING GO

What would change in your experience of mothering if you did not have to be perfect? Where are you being hard on yourself? What could you let yourself off the hook for? What stops you from letting yourself off the hook?

Give yourself permission to change your mind. The way you thought you would do things may be different from how you want to do them now, after you've met your baby and gotten to know him or her.

Mothering that comes from a place of connection to ourselves and to our children leads us to a deeper sense of calm and true responsibility. Just as each child is unique in his or her needs, so is each mother, and when we listen to and are aligned with our own values, our children feel that. It's worth it even if you need to fight to hear your own voice. There is no one who knows what is better for your child than you do.

Motherhood isn't a process to experience alone; it is a transition of becoming that requires sisterhood and witnesses. We need to be able to express the depth of our feelings to someone who can listen and understand without trying to fix anything, talk us out of how we feel, or help us see the bright side. Finding your own voice and following what it says becomes easier when that voice is not just echoing around inside your head. Surrounded by wise women and loving elders who have had their own challenges and triumphs helps to illuminate the ordinariness of those choices that easily become weighty.

You, as yourself, need to find your own counsel of wise women, whether that is by seeking professional help, by reaching out to a network of friends and family, or both. You, as mother, need a multiplicity of mother figures—*todas las madres*—as does your child. Clarissa Pinkola Estés, author of *Women Who Run with the Wolves*, said to her own daughter: "You are born with one mother, but if you are lucky you will have more than one. And among them all, you will find most of what you need."

Identify the women in your life who have mothered you or who you would like to mother you. Reach out to them so that you feel supported and mothered as you become a mother. Know that by doing so, not only will you enrich your child's life, your own life, and your family life, but you will also stitch back together part of the torn fabric of community that we are all longing for.

When we ask for help and allow support to come from many directions, we model trust in life. We demonstrate the knowing that things are fundamentally okay. We widen the real net of interconnectedness. We contribute to the true legacy that we wish to continue.

YOUR LEGACY

....

Write a letter to your baby about what your process of giving birth and becoming a mother has been like. Tell your child what you wish you would have known. Give her the gift of your experience. Offer your advice about how she can take care of herself, her partner, and her children—your grandchildren. Light the way for your family.

SUMMARY

- Your relationship to your mother is a fundamental piece of your psychological and physical health and is especially awakened when you become a mother.
- Becoming a good enough mother means that you can let go of perfection and know that good mothering is about the quality of the repair that is made after there are mistakes. Modeling making mistakes and then repairing them is a valuable part of mothering.
- You do not have to love every part of parenting.
- Reach out to other women to help mother you as you continue on your own journey into motherhood.

Reflections
- What parts of mothering have surprised you?
- What do you genuinely dislike or even hate about mothering?
- What do you enjoy about mothering?
- What would change in your experience of mothering if you did not have to be perfect?
- Where are you being hard on yourself?
- What could you let yourself off the hook for?
- What stops you from letting yourself off the hook?

Exercises

- Learn to listen to your intuition by tuning in to your body, using the body compass.
- Write out some of the edicts you've been told by others about how to mother your baby and then respond to them honestly, to tap into your intuition through journaling.
- Write your mother a letter from you as mother. Write your mother a letter from you as the child. Keep them in your journal, or burn them to release the words into the universe.
- Make a mother lineage tree.
- Write a letter to your baby.

Conclusion:

CONTINUING
THE REVOLUTION

.... 🌿 ....

And so it is that the one who rocks the cradle
of the babe is the one who holds up the lamp,
shedding light on the world.
—MATA AMRITANANDAMAYI

At the beginning of this book, I wrote about the Postpartum Revolution and the time that we live in. The truth is, progress—whether it be cultural, political, spiritual, or individual—is not a straight line. It dips up and down and can sometimes feel like we're taking one step forward just to take two steps back. And that's okay, whether you are feeling that way about your own progress or our culture's. The main thing is that you keep at it.

What does that mean? It means the Postpartum Revolution is now in your hands—in every woman's (and hopefully her partner's) hands. It's time for you to take your own torch and light the way for others. When you began this journey of birth and motherhood, you looked to me—to this book—to help light your way. When you had questions, you looked for answers. When you wanted to find tools that could help you, you searched them out. My greatest hope for you is that as you journey beyond the fourth trimester, you not only continue to seek out the tools, help, and community, including postpartum doulas, bodyworkers, doctors, and friends and family, for support when you need it, but also offer it as well. Sharing your experience—both the challenges that you worked through and the elements of early mothering that were easier than you thought—is what will create the open dialogue we need so that less women feel like they are in the dark and unnecessarily surprised when they join the journey. It is not only knowledge that will reach across the bridge to the new mother, warmth, heart, and solidarity will reach her too and let her know that this time is challenging by nature—but she is not alone.

The fourth trimester is one of the most important opportunities in a new mother's life to instill long-term health and to set herself and her family up for a lifetime of optimal health and bonding. And right now, this period of time sits at a unique cultural crossroads.

We have a chance to move toward real community and interdependence, where instead of hoarding resources, we share them with one another. We have the chance to step into a new feminism that honors women's bodies, not just our reproductive rights, but also our unique access to the wisdom that living with monthly cycles and blood rites offers. We can live into a new wave of feminism that has space for women's embodiment and pleasure, one where we celebrate ourselves and are celebrated for our own inherent worth, rather than running ourselves ragged trying to "do it all."

You now have the knowledge, the tools, and a torch of your own to help light the way.

acknowledgments

·········· ❦ ··········

There are a few people who have been with this book from preconception to birth. Without them, this book would have been frozen in time, left behind at any number of stages.

A special thanks to Joelle Hann, a friend and editor so true that she came from New York to Rio to ferret out a form from all my ideas and experiences and to make sure I got the proposal done. She assured me and reassured me that I was the one to write this book, and that even in the face of single parenting and freelance work, I could do it. She never lost sight of the purpose of this book for the lives of women and mothers, and championed me at every doubting turn.

It takes a village to raise a child. It takes a village to raise a mother. And it takes a village to write a book. I was able to write this book because for the first time since becoming a mother, I finally had the support that I suggest every mother needs to thrive. My parents gave me every type of support possible—a place to live, emergency school pick-ups, long weekends away, and pep talks. Mom: you gave me life, and you have given this book a life through your presence in Cecilia's. Dad: thank you for being my first model of the masculine in service to the feminine, and for showing that to Cece. Thank you for believing in me.

Thank you to my dearest friends who had lengthy conversations with me, who stepped up to care for Cecilia, who asked me how it was going, who shared their own experiences of motherhood, and who believed in this work throughout the process. These women are each so profound in their own right that this book is as much theirs as it is mine: Heather Rowley, Ruthie Fraser, Ellen Boeder, Chrisandra Fox, Lindsay Mackay Ashmun, Erin Harper, Maggie Rintala, Paula Self, Laura Regalbuto, and Fernanda Pinheiro.

To my Brazilian friend-family, who cradled me and helped me grow as a woman and a mother, never judging and always loving: Jenny, Helcio, Vivi, Sergio, Fernanda, Stefano, Ale, Lis, Paula, and Greice.

I had the special counsel from a group of wise women and single mothers when we convened as a quartet: Alison Marie, Jennifer Owens, and Centehua Sage. Their support happened on all realms, seen and unseen to bring this work forward.

Also in my cosmic support corner at all times were Ash Robinson, Maura Rassman, Sue Glumac, and Monisha Chandanani, whose wisdom is sprinkled in nonlinear ways throughout.

Taylor Phinny and Laura Centorrino shared their sorcery in helping me understand the energy dimensions more deeply. Eden Fromberg, MD, consulted on various sections of this book, setting me straight and offering her decades of wisdom bridging the worlds of holistic healing and Western medicine. Conversations with acupuncturists and scholars Micah Arsham, Kristin Hauser, Kristin Gonzalez, and Sabine Wilms made sure that I honored the Chinese medicine tradition. Bhakti Wong also contributed her vast experience in yogic arts, bodywork, and traditional Asian postpartum healing traditions—this book is enriched by her sweetness. Cristal Mortensen was instrumental in the development of all the sections on how to work with the nervous system in a practical way. She also was there at the pivotal moments when I needed soul strengthening. Ellen Boeder's friendship and deep insight as a mother and a relationship counselor enriches everything on intimacy and relationship.

To my Magamama team, Centehua and Maria: thanks for believing in this mission and being pioneers. And Centehua, this book is enriched a thousand-fold by your food-medicine wisdom and kitchen magic.

To Heloisa Lessa and Maysa Luduvice Gomez: thank you for your care and the gift of my birth as a mother. I have learned so much from both of you.

All of the employees at Lofty Coffee met me with smiles, checked in on my progress, and helped make writing this book all the more enjoyable with great coffee.

To all my teachers of yoga, Rolfing, Somatic Experiencing, and Sexological Bodywork, my auspicious karma in these departments is not lost on me, and I am using every ounce of wisdom that I gleaned for the healing of all beings.

To all the women who have blessed me by sharing your stories, your lives, and your bodies with me to explore the kaleidoscopic reality of this work. To Robin Lim, Aviva Romm, Christiane Northrup, Maya Tiwari, Jeannine Parvati Baker, Tami Lynn Kent, Pam England, Uma Dinsmore-Tuli, Ina May Gaskin, and Tsultrim Allione, who stood as beacons—mothers, visionaries, healers, and advocates of women everywhere, on your shoulders I stand. Thank you for showing me a way. To Alisa Vitti, whose book was a salvation and who then graciously accepted my invitation to write the foreword for this book.

Thanks to Beth Frankl for seeing the value in this work immediately, and to the whole team at Shambhala Publications for creating such a beautiful book. Thank you, Wren, for bringing the illustrations to life, with beauty and true artistry. Thanks to Gretchen Stelter for bringing the finish line back into sight.

And finally, to my mentor Ellen Heed, who showed me this road to healing for myself and for the thousands of women we now serve. I owe my full recovery and radiant health that has become the platform for my life's work, as well as the eyes to see this path, to you.

KIMBERLY ANN JOHNSON

Appendix 1:
POSTPARTUM SANCTUARY PLAN

....

The postpartum time is a period of great change on every level—physical, mental, emotional, sexual, and spiritual. This postpartum plan will help you to build a foundation so that you can attend to the five universal postpartum needs: rest, nourishing food, loving touch, companionship, and contact with nature.

VISITORS

Who do you want to visit in the first three days?

_____

In the first two weeks?

_____

In the first month?

_____

REST

What do you anticipate might be obstacles to resting for you?

_____

What are ways that you can address those?

_____

How will you create the space to nap during the day?

_____

How will you manage visitors to ensure space for resting? (See Sign for Your Front Door in appendix 4 for ideas.)

_____

How will you manage technology (devices, mobile phone, computers)? When will you unplug?

_____

FOOD

List three of your favorite and most nourishing meals. (You can also see recipes in appendix 6 for ideas.)

_____

List three balanced snacks that you love.

_____

Who can organize the meal train?

_____

Include dietary needs and restrictions for your family for the meal train.

_____

Assemble takeout menus. Which restaurants deliver?

_____

COMPANIONSHIP

Gather Your Tribe

Think about your tribe, the people who you know are there for you, and that you can trust for emotional support or to lend a helping hand. Fill in names and phone numbers to make it one step easier when the time comes and you need them!

Who can you call to tell how you are really feeling about mothering and who will listen without judgment or advice?

_____

Who could you call if you want to take a shower and need someone to hold your baby?

_____

Who would you trust to take your baby for a walk?

_____

Who can you talk to about the hard mothering decisions that you feel would be safe and would not judge you?

_____

Who do you know who makes wholesome and nutritious food?

_____

Who could you call if you want someone to sit with you and hang out?

_____

Who do you know whose mothering you respect?

_____

Who would you like weekly visits from?

_____

Who is knowledgeable about local contacts for health care?

_____

Your Wider Tribe of Wellness Support

Now think about your wider tribe—the people that you can assemble to provide you with self-care expertise, wellness information, and expert care, when needed. Put this list on the refrigerator so that when you need the resource it is easy to find.

Somatic therapist

Holistic pelvic care/scar-tissue remediation specialist

Lactation consultant

Chiropractor

Massage therapist

Acupuncturist

Ob-gyn

Midwife

Housekeeper

Postpartum doula

Night nurse

Local breastfeeding support group

Local playgroups

Mommy and me exercise groups

WHAT BRINGS YOU JOY

Now that you know your body will be nourished and you have your tribe on-call, how will your mind and spirit be nourished? When you feel a little off, what gets you back on track? Here are some ideas. Make this list your own. Write it out on a Post-it or in lipstick on your mirror to remind yourself of the little things that you love.

Singing
Music
Movement
Reading inspirational words
Watching great films
Talking with a dear friend

Make a list of audiobooks, uplifting shows, and podcasts that interest you. Download them so that they are ready to listen to during long nursing stretches.

_____

_____

_____

_____

_____

_____

_____

_____

_____

_____

_____

_____

_____

_____

Appendix 2A:
POSTPARTUM RELATIONSHIP PLAN

....

With some simple communication, you can set your relationship up for success after having a baby. Make two copies and fill them out separately. Then compare your answers and use them to form a plan to stay connected during this time of change. Refer to chapter 3 for more in-depth explanation of these questions.

What is your love language?

_____

What is your partner's love language?

_____

How do you deal with stress?

_____

How does your partner deal with stress?

_____

How do you recognize that stress in each other?

_____

How can you help each other cope with that stress when it's happening?

_____

What can you ask each other for now that you can refer to later?

_____

What do you commit to in your relationship once you have a baby?

_____

Establish your plan for daily three to five minute check-ins. (When will you do these?) How will you remind each other?

_____

_____

_____

_____

_____

Appendix 2B:
DIVIDING HOUSEHOLD CHORES

....

I borrowed this practical exercise from Elly Taylor's book, *Becoming Us*. When a new baby comes, the little things around the house add up. For some new moms, it's very hard to relax when things seem like they are falling apart and chaotic around the house. This exercise lets you decide what is essential—what absolutely has to get done—what is preferable, and what is forgettable. This will help to keep things in perspective, guide you to choose what you absolutely need to hire help for, and what you can let go of for a while.

Make a list of all the chores that normally need doing around the home: including caring for older children, laundry, trash, plant watering, dog walking, and so on. Work out which ones are essential (E), preferable (P) and forgettable (F). Then work out who is going to do what, keeping in mind it's easy to overestimate and overextend, and the main priority is nesting and resting. Outsource what you can and be willing to negotiate everything as mama's, baby's, and dad's or partner's needs change over the next few months.

_____

_____

_____

_____

_____

_____

_____

_____

_____

_____

_____

_____

_____

Appendix 3:

LETTER FOR
MEAL TRAIN PARTICIPANTS

....

Dear _____,

Thank you so much for contributing to our meal train. This is going to be one of the most nourishing and supportive gifts that you could give. We are grateful for whatever you are offering, and to make it a little easier for you, here are some suggestions.

Midwives suggest five days on the bed, five days in the bed, and five days around the bed, so mama and baby will be lying in for those first three weeks.

After that, we would love to have fifteen to twenty minute visits. If you could help the new mama with that, it would be great. She will probably get excited and want to talk more, but she needs help remembering to prioritize rest.

Three meals I love are:

_____

_____

_____

Foods that are not favorites/that I don't like:

_____

My favorite foods are:

_____

I have allergies to:

_____

Thank you so much for your support at this special time.

With great love and appreciation,

Appendix 4:

SIGN FOR
YOUR FRONT DOOR

....

When you are tired, overwhelmed or recovering, it can be difficult to find the right words. Here is are some things you could put on a sign to post on the front door or in your kitchen.

Thank you visiting us and welcoming our little love!

A short stay is the perfect gift, supporting both nurture and rest.

Your love and help—in ways big and small—are so welcome!

Lending a hand could be washing the dishes, checking the laundry, or making sure we've had a snack. Mama also might like a hot bath or a long hug.

Appendix 5:
ESSENTIAL FOODS
FOR POSTPARTUM HEALING

....

The information on food in this book is influenced by the principles of Ayurveda and Chinese medicine, as well as the legacy of the Weston Price foundation with the understanding that animal fats and cholesterol are vital factors for the nourishment of the brain and nervous system.

Many whole foods are appropriate for the postpartum time. What foods you choose will vary depending on what is available locally and in season. Below is a list of foods that are especially antioxidant, blood building, and mineral rich. All over the world, postpartum foods share these qualities of nutrient density. The preparation during the postpartum phase is of vital importance. In general, food should be warm and oily (naturally saturated, or covered in fats like ghee, butter, and lard). They should also be prepared with the right spices to help keep a mother's inner body warm, aid digestion, and stimulate the circulatory system.

A well-stocked pantry will ensure that you have the raw ingredients you need to make healthy, nourishing meals and snacks, instead of defaulting to easy fast food options, at a time when nutrition is paramount to your long-term health. What follows is a sample pantry list.

FRUITS AND VEGETABLES

In essence, all vegetables and fruits are of benefit. However some of them are especially powerful antioxidants. How they are prepared is also important. Lightly steaming vegetables and stewing fruits when possible is helpful for digestion at this time.

Avocados: An excellent source for polyunsaturated and monounsaturated fat, which help the body absorb fat soluble vitamins that feed the brain and assist the nervous system.

Bananas: Rich in potassium, vitamin B^6, vitamin C, manganese, fiber, and protein, this fruit also moderates blood sugar levels and aids the digestive system.

Beets: With essential nutrients such as B vitamins, magnesium, boron, and iron, beets are blood builders, and they balance cholesterol levels and help maintain a healthy cardiovascular system.

Blueberries (and other berries): Berries are loaded with fiber, manganese, vitamin K, and vitamin C. They are an extremely high antioxidant food, helping the body neutralize free radicals and repair DNA damage.

Cherry tomatoes: A great source for vitamin C, vitamin A, and B^6. They may help repair cellular damage and protect against osteoporosis and skin damage.

Dandelion greens: Rich in Vitamin B complex as well as minerals such as choline, magnesium, boron, and iron. These can also aid the digestive system, liver, and gallbladder.

Figs: This stone fruit will help lower high blood pressure and they are loaded with potassium, essential minerals, and high density of phenolic antioxidants. They protect the heart and regulate kidney and liver functions.

Mango: The most effective antioxidant, mangoes are loaded with vitamin C, pectin, and fiber. They help to lower serum cholesterol levels and boost the immune system and are alkalizing to the whole body due to the content of tartaric acid, malic acid, and citric acid.

Papaya: Containing papain, an enzyme that helps digest proteins, papayas are loaded with antioxidants such as vitamin C, flavonoids, vitamin B, folate, and pantothenic acid, which help reduce inflammation.

Passion fruit: Rich in potassium, vitamin C, and minerals, including magnesium and iron, passion fruit is also an excellent antioxidant and helps regulate heart rate and blood pressure.

Pears: These are mineral rich in magnesium, folate, calcium, and iron, as well as high in vitamin C and fiber, which aids the digestive system.

Persimmon: An excellent antioxidant and a source for beta-carotene and vitamin C, this fruit also contains compounds that are anti-inflammatory and anti-hemorrhagic. They are rich in minerals, including copper, which helps build red blood cells.

Pomegranate: A great source for vitamin B complex, minerals, vitamin C, and antioxidants, pomegranates also improve circulation and help build immunity.

NUTS, SEEDS, AND GRAINS

All nuts, seeds, and grains should be soaked for a minimum of one hour (or you can just leave them overnight) to make them easier to digest and to awaken the nutrients, making them bio-available.

Nuts

Almonds: Protein rich, almonds contain calcium and manganese and are also anti-inflammatory.

Cashews: These nuts are rich in vitamin E and K, selenium, antioxidants, and minerals.

Walnuts: These nuts contain essential fatty acids, protein, and minerals.

Seeds

Cacao nibs: An excellent source of magnesium, an essential mineral for the respiratory and circulatory system, as well as a source of essential minerals and phytonutrients.

Chia seeds: These are the most bio-available protein source, helping the body stay hydrated and moisturized from within.

Hemp seeds: These seeds contain omega fatty acids, protein, and fiber, as well as having anti-inflammatory and antioxidant properties.

Millet: This seed is rich in protein, fiber, and minerals, helping to regulate blood sugars.

Pumpkin seeds: These are mineral rich, as well as having antioxidant and anti-inflammatory properties.

Sunflower seeds: Full of protein, this good carbohydrate is also a mineral rich choice.

Grains

Amaranth: This grain is protein rich as well as filled with fiber and other important phytonutrients, including the amino acid lysine.

Quinoa: This grain is protein rich, full of fiber, and has anti-inflammatory and antioxidant properties.

Wild rice blend or brown rice: These types of rice are full of protein, fiber, and good carbohydrates.

BEVERAGES AND LIQUIDS

Cow's milk is not on this list because the proteins are large and difficult to digest for both mother and baby, unless it is raw and unpasteurized. Minimize carbonated drinks and caffeine because they are dehydrating. Herbal teas are a great substitute and can have medicinal value, while contributing to hydration of the tissues.

Almond milk

Oat milk

Hemp milk

Fennel tea

Chamomile tea

Raspberry leaf tea

Roasted dandelion tea

Rooibos tea

FATS

Now is a time to consider fats as a vital role in your healing process and overall health and well-being of your entire family. Fats are vital for proper brain function and absorbing nutrients, which is why we feel good when eating healthy fats.

All good for you, the difference is in fat composition. For example, olive oil is mostly monounsaturated as is lard (yes, lard) while coconut oil is mostly saturated, as is ghee. As with all things, sourcing is the major concern. Whether choosing duck fat, beef tallow, butter, olive oil, avocado, or coconut oil, you want to source the highest quality possible. It is of essential value to choose pastured and 100 percent grass-fed animal fats, for the health and quality of life of the animal is immediately translated into your health.

> Olive oil (not for cooking)
> Coconut oil
> Ghee
> Butter
> Lard

PROTEINS

When choosing proteins, whether plant-based or animal-based, it's important to source the highest quality possible. Our foods are being mass-produced which, comes with a whole set of issues including the use of toxic pesticides and hormones. It is vital to support farmers and companies who raise animals and grow food at a smaller scale with ethical, sustainable, and humane practices and to eliminate the ingestion of unnecessary toxins. If choosing plant-based proteins also look for fair trade products or buy directly from farmers when possible. Plant-based proteins include beans, lentils, grains, and hemp products, which are among the most bio-available protein sources and are rich in Omega 3 and 6 fatty acids.

If choosing fish, I highly recommend looking for sustainable companies who line catch wild fish. Farm raised fish is usually fed GM feed and added color.

I recommend choosing 100 percent grass-fed animal products, pastured chicken, dairy, and eggs.

Animal Proteins

Bone broth

Chicken breasts or thighs

Ground beef/buffalo

Turkey sausage

Duck

Bacon

Salmon

Raw cheese

Full fat yogurt

Cottage cheese

Kefir

Plant Proteins

Hemp seeds

Chia seeds

Spirulina

Red lentils

Mung beans

Chickpeas

Amaranth

Quinoa

SWEETENERS

Postpartum, low glycemic index and stable blood sugar levels will help your hormones recalibrate. Here are some options for natural sweeteners.

Local raw honey: Honey contains essential nutrients and is a medicine. It is also important to support small scale local beekeepers that ensure ethical care and natural practices. Local honey is a natural antibiotic and is anti-fungal and anti-viral.

Maple syrup: Mineral rich and low glycemic, this is a perfect choice for a sweetener.

Yacon syrup: Made from the yacon root, this syrup is mineral rich and low glycemic, high in antioxidants and potassium. It can help regulate blood sugar levels.

EASY SNACKS

These are balanced nutrient-rich, high-fat snacks that nourish brain and nervous system function.

Rye crisps with nut butter, ghee, avocado, or raw cheese
Dried figs or dried apricots with raw cheese
Medjool dates with ghee or almond butter
Nori with tahini and banana
Raw trail mix
Full fat yogurt with fruit and seeds
Cottage cheese and fruit

Appendix 6:
RECIPES

....

These are a few simple, nutrient-dense staple recipes to give you a start in your postpartum repertoire. For more guidance and delicious recipes, visit: www.magamama.com/fourthtrimesterrecipes.

MINERAL-RICH NUT BAR

This sweet treat is nutrient dense and comforting. Loaded with essential fatty acids, B^{12}, protein, magnesium, selenium, and fiber.

MAKES ABOUT 4 BARS

½ cup cashews

½ cup Brazil nuts (soaked overnight or for a couple of hours)

1⅓ cups macademia nuts (soaked and dried)

3 tablespoons hemps seeds

5 to 6 dates (medjool, pitted)

2 tablespoons pastured organic ghee or coconut oil

½ teaspoon Ashitaba powder

⅓ teaspoon cinnamon

Pinch each of Himalayan salt, nutmeg, cardamom

1. Place the nuts and hemp seeds in a food processor and crush until the mix resembles flour.
2. Add the dates, ghee or coconut oil, Ashitaba, salt, and spices, and process until the mixture comes together like dough.
3. Wrap up the dough in parchment paper and shape it into a large bar.
4. Keep the bar in the fridge and slice as desired.

MOTHER'S MILK ELIXIR

An elixir is a drink that targets a specific need often using herbal medicine. This mother's milk herbal blend is a lactagogue that promotes milk production and is rich in iron that helps build blood.

MAKES 2 CUPS

> 2 cups water
>
> Fennel, nettle, rose, and raspberry-leaf tea blend
>
> 1 teaspoon almond butter
>
> 1 teaspoon raw honey
>
> Pinch of cinnamon

1. Boil the water and steep the herbal infusion for 3 to 5 minutes.
2. Pour the infusion into the blender—reserving the herbs—with the almond butter, honey, and cinnamon. Make sure that there is an opening on the blender lid for steam to escape.
3. Blend on low and gradually increase the speed until the mixture is frothy.
4. Pour into a heatproof mug and enjoy immediately.
5. You can reuse the herbs for a lighter tea, simply add more boiled water and let it steep.

AMARANTH MORNING PORRIDGE

This is a nutrient dense and comforting meal. Amaranth is a native staple food in Central and South America and has been cultivated for thousands of years due to its extraordinary nourishing qualities. It's rich in essential minerals such as manganese, calcium, iron, fiber, and the amino acid lysine, which helps absorb calcium and produce energy. A great source for bio-available plant protein and other phytonutrients.

SERVES 4

>   3 cups amaranth
>   1 cup raw milk or nut milk
>   ⅓ cup crushed nuts
>   ⅓ cup goji berries
>   ⅓ cup blackberries, or your favorite berry
>   1 tablespoon ghee
>   1 tablespoon maple syrup

1. Soak the amaranth in 9 cups (2 liters) of water overnight.
2. Pour the amaranth and soaking water into a pot. Bring to a boil and simmer for 20 minutes, or until soft.
3. Add the milk, nuts, berries, ghee, and maple syrup. The amounts could vary per your preference.
4. Other toppings you could try are chia seeds, hemp seeds, and shredded coconut.

NETTLE BONE BROTH

This is a highly nourishing food at any time of day. It's important to choose 100 percent grass-fed animal bones to ensure quality and preferably wild harvested nettles, but nettle tea found in bulk works too. Nettles are high in iron, which helps build blood and nourish the cells. Bone broth mineralizes the body and is rich in essential fatty acids, which nourish the nervous system and assist the gut flora. If you don't have nettles, you can substitute spinach.

SERVES 6 TO 8

3 pounds of bones from a healthy pastured animal (cow, sheep, chicken, or turkey)

½ leek, roughly chopped

1 small celery root, peeled and roughly chopped

2 carrots, roughly chopped

1 onion, roughly chopped

4 whole garlic cloves

2 tablespoons apple cider vinegar

1 tablespoon lard or coconut oil

2 large bunches of wild stinging nettles—optional (if available for harvest or found at farmers markets)

1 sprig rosemary

1 bunch parsley or cilantro

3 culinary sage leaves

2 bay leaves

1 tablespoon Himalayan salt

1 teaspoon peppercorns

1. Preheat oven to 450°F.
2. Place the bones, leek, celery root, carrots, onion, and garlic cloves in a roasting pan and coat them with the apple cider vinegar and the lard or oil. Roast for 20 minutes.
3. Toss the ingredients and roast for another 20 minutes for flavor, and so the bones begin to release the fats.
4. After roasting, pour 13 cups of spring water in a 6-quart stockpot and add the nettles, herbs, salt, and peppercorns. Add the roasted bones and vegetables and add more water if the bones and vegetables are not fully submerged.
5. Cover the pot and bring the contents to a gentle boil. Then, reduce the heat to low and simmer with the lid slightly ajar for at least 8 hours. The longer it simmers, the better it gets. Continue to adjust water as needed to ensure bones and vegetables are submerged, occasionally skimming off excess foam and fat.
6. Remove the pot from the heat and let it cool slightly. Strain out all the ingredients with a fine mesh sieve, reserving only the broth, and adjust the salt as desired and enjoy. You can drink the broth as is, and it also may be used in other dishes, like rice, quinoa, or as a base for soups. A couple ounces with each meal will aid digestion. The bones may be used for another round of broth as well. Keep adding water and more herbs for flavor in new batches.
7. Keep the broth in the fridge in small containers. Once chilled, a layer of fat will solidify on top; simply scrape off this layer before pouring to reheat on stove. This broth keeps well for 5 days in the fridge or 4 months in the freezer.

HEART-WARMING CACAO

Nutrient rich hot chocolate is highly mineralizing and contains protein, essential fatty acids, and omega 3 and 6 oils. This is feel-good food that is also nourishing and calming to the nervous system. Shatavari is part of the asparagus family and is commonly used in Ayurvedic medicine to rejuvenate women's reproductive systems. It also soothes to the digestive tract, helps regulate hormones, and promotes healthy milk production.

Cacao paste is rich in the essential mineral magnesium; cacao is highly supportive to the cardiovascular and respiratory systems, and promotes feelings of well-being through the help of the fatty-acid neurotransmitters anandamide and PEA, also known as the bliss chemicals.

Cacao in its pure raw form is a medicine and is not overstimulating to the nervous system. It is actually soothing and warming, reduces inflammation, and boosts mood.

SERVES 4

> 3 cups spring water
>
> ⅓ cup raw cacao paste (available from longevitywarehouse.com)
>
> 2 tablespoons raw honey
>
> 1 teaspoon cinnamon
>
> 1 pinch nutmeg
>
> 2 tablespoons hemp seeds
>
> 1 teaspoon Shatavari powder (available from mountainroseherbs.com)

1. Bring the water to a gentle boil in a medium saucepan.
2. Put all the ingredients in a high-powered blender and pour in the hot water. Blend the mixture slowly on low, ensuring that there is an opening on the lid for steam to escape.
3. Gradually increase the blender speed to medium and then high, until the hemp seeds are dissolved and the elixir is frothy.
4. Adjust honey to taste and enjoy immediately. This will keep in the fridge for 2 days.

NO-CAFFEINE CHAI

This tasty beverage contains the benefits of the warming herbs and spices without the caffeine.

I enjoy rooibos or chamomile for this recipe. These herbs and spices aid the digestive fires, stimulate the circulatory system, and keep the body warm. You can also double the recipe for a larger batch and keep it in the fridge for 3 to 4 days.

SERVES 4

⅓ cup water

2 cups raw pastured milk or your favorite nut milk

1 teaspoon loose rooibos or any other desired tea

3 pieces of cinnamon bark

2 inches fresh ginger

3 cardamom pods

2 cloves

¼ teaspoon fennel seeds

1 pinch nutmeg (freshly grated)

2 tablespoons raw local honey

1. Add the water, milk, and all of the dry spices to a medium saucepan (leaving the honey out).
2. Bring the mixture to a gentle boil and then reduce the heat. Stir constantly with a wooden spoon so the milk does not burn on the bottom of pan.
3. Simmer for 15 minutes.
4. Remove the chai from the heat, strain it with a fine mesh sieve, add the honey to taste, and enjoy immediately.

NETTLE PESTO

Nettles are potent medicine, their exceptional iron content helps build blood and restore balance in the bodies of new mamas. Hemp seeds are protein rich and contain essential fatty acids including omega 3s and 6s. However if fresh nettles are not available, simply substitute with any greens—spinach, sorrel, cilantro, mustard, or others. Pesto is an easy and delicious way to add extra nutrients to any dish. I like dropping a dollop in soups, on meat or fish, or over rice and other grains.

SERVES 6 TO 8

> 1 large bunch stinging nettles
> 1 bunch basil
> ½ bunch parsley
> ⅓ cup raw cashews (soaked for 20 minutes)
> 2 tablespoons hemp seeds
> 1 garlic clove
> 1 cup unfiltered olive oil
> 1 teaspoon Himalayan salt
> Pinch of pepper

1. Put all of the ingredients in a high-powered blender and adjust the oil if needed to achieve desired consistency.
2. Taste and adjust salt and serve immediately. This can be stored in the fridge for up to 6 days.

bibliography

.... ❀ ....

Allione, Tsultrim. *Women of Wisdom*. Boston, MA: Snow Lion,
2000.

Brizendine, Louann. *The Female Brain*. New York: Morgan Road
Books, 2006.

Brogan, Kelly. *A Mind of Your Own: The Truth About Depression and
How Women Can Heal Their Bodies to Reclaim their Lives*. New
York: Harper Wave, 2016.

Calais-Germain, Blandine. *The Female Pelvis Anatomy & Exercises*.
Seattle: Eastland Press, 2003.

Chapman, Gary. *The 5 Love Languages: The Secrets to Love that
Lasts*. Chicago: Northfield Publishing, 2015. (Fifth Edition)

Dinsmore-Tuli, Uma. *Yoni Shakti: A Woman's Guide to Power and
Freedom through Yoga and Tantra*. London: YogaWords, 2014.

Dunham, Carroll. *Mamatoto: A Celebration of Birth*. London:
Viking, 2001.

England, Pam. *Ancient Map for Modern Birth*. Albuquerque, NM:
Seven Gates Media, 2017.

England, Pam and Horowitz, Rob. *Birthing from Within: An
Extra-Ordinary Guide to Childbirth Preparation*. Albuquerque,
NM: Partera Press, 1998.

Ensler, Eve. *In the Body of the World: A Memoir of Cancer and Connection*. New York: Metropolitan Books, 2013.

Fallon, Sally. *Nourishing Traditions: The Cookbook that Challenges
Politically Correct Nutrition and Diet Dictocrats*. Washington, DC:
New Trends Publishing, 2001. (Revised Second Edition)

Gutman, Laura. *Maternity: Coming Face to Face with Your Own
Shadow*. Albuquerque, NM: Crianza USA, 2002.

Herrera, Isa. *Ending Female Pain: A Woman's Manual*. New York:
Duplex, 2014. (Second Edition)

Hulme, Janet A. *Solving the Mystery of the Pelvic Rotator Cuff: Back Pain, Balance, Bladder and Bowel Health*. Peoria, IL: Phoenix Publishing Group, 2005.

Jordan, Brigitte and Davis-Floyd, Robbie. *Birth in Four Cultures: A Crosscultural Investigation of Childbirth in Yucatan, Holland, Sweden, and the United States*. Long Grove, IL: Waveland Press, 1992. (Fourth Edition)

Kent, Tami Lynn. *Mothering from Your Center: Tapping Your Body's Natural Energy for Pregnancy, Birth, and Parenting*. New York: Atria/Beyond Words, 2013.

——. *Wild Feminine: Finding Power, Spirit & Joy in the Female Body*. New York: Atria/Beyond Words, 2011.

Levine, Peter A. *Waking the Tiger: Healing Trauma*. Berkeley, CA: North Atlantic Books, 1997.

Lim, Robin. *After the Baby's Birth: A Woman's Way to Wellness: A Complete Guide for Postpartum Women*. Berkeley, CA: Celestial Arts, 1995.

McNamara, Brooke. *Feed Your Vow, Poems for Falling Into Fullness*. Boulder: Performance Integral, 2015.

Miller, Karen Maezen. *Momma Zen: Walking the Crooked Path of Motherhood*. Boston: Trumpeter, 2006.

Northrup, Christiane. *Mother-Daughter Wisdom: Understanding the Crucial Link Between Mothers, Daughters, and Health*. New York: Bantam Dell, 2006.

Ou, Heng, Marisa Belger, and Amely Greeven. *The First Forty Days: The Essential Art of Nourishing the New Mother*. New York: Stewart, Tabori & Chang, 2016.

Pitchford, Paul. *Healing with Whole Foods: Asian Traditions and Modern Nutrition*. California: North Atlantic Books, 2003. (Third Edition)

Rolf, Ida P. *Rolfing: Reestablishing the Natural Alignment and Structural Integration of the Human Body for Vitality and Well-Being*.

Rochester, VT: Healing Arts Press, 1989. (Revised Edition)

Romm, Aviva Jill. *Natural Health after Birth: The Complete Guide to Postpartum Wellness*. Rochester, VT: Healing Arts Press, 2002.

Taylor, Elly. *Becoming Us: 8 Steps to Grow a Family that Thrives*. Sydney, Australia: Three Turtles Press, 2014.

Tiwari, Maya. *Women's Power to Heal: Through Inner Medicine*. Mount Penn, PA: Mother Om Media, 2012.

Van Gennep, Arnold. *The Rites of Passage*. Chicago: University of Chicago Press, 1960.

Vitti, Alisa. *WomanCode: Perfect Your Cycle, Amplify Your Fertility, Supercharge Your Sex Drive, and Become a Power Source*. New York: HarperOne, 2013.

Vopni, Kim. *Prepare to Push*. Vancouver, BC: Pelvienne Wellness, 2014.

Welsh, Claudia. *Balance Your Hormones, Balance Your Life: Achieving Optimal Health and Wellness through Ayurveda, Chinese Medicine, and Western Science*. Cambridge, MA: Da Capo Lifelong Books, 2011.

Wertz, Richard W., and Wertz, Dorothy C. *Lying In: A History of Childbirth in America*. New York: The Free Press, 1977.

Winston, Sheri. *Women's Anatomy of Arousal*. Kingston, NY: Mango Garden Press, 2009.

Zhao, Xiaolan. *Reflections of the Moon on Water: Healing Women's Bodies and Minds through Traditional Chinese Wisdom*. Toronto, ON: Random House Canada, 2006.

index

Page numbers in italics refer to pages that also have illustrations.

birth injuries, 1, 174, 200
  causes of, difficulties in identifying, 177
  grieving, 290
  painful periods after, 195
  sexuality and, 258, 271–72, 274, 275
  statistics on, 219
birth rehearsals, 56–57, 80
birth stories
  for births that need healing, 219–21
  importance of, 209, 225
  narrating, 211–13
  nonwritten ways of telling, 216
  of partners, 235–37, 242
  power of, 216–17
  writing exercise, 212–13
Birth Story Medicine, 17, 221, 275
birth trauma, 87–88, 226
  healing, 217–18, 219
  professional help for, 221–22
  sexuality and, 275
blood
  Ayurvedic view of, 130–31
  bleeding after childbirth, 195–96
  deficiencies, 142
  foods for building, 124–25
  improving circulation of, 138
  sugar levels in, maintaining, 180
blood work, 116, 117, 118, 180
body, physical
  after childbirth, 145–46
  awareness of, 66
  cellular memory of, 105–6
  connection with one's own, 9–10,
    146–47
  intelligence of, 177
  internal environment of, 179–80
  learning to love, 248–50
  listening to, 66, 68, 256, 258
  reclaiming, 138
  as ritual sacrifice, 205
  self-regulation of, 37
  sensing, exercise for, 280–81
  sexual identity and, 268
  See also spiritual body
body dysmorphia, 10
BodyMind Centering, 106
body-mind connection, 10
bodywork, 4, 172

for babies, 106
benefits of, 166–67
need for, 30
for pelvic floor, 81, 98
sexological, 186, 257
types of, 167–70
types to avoid, 168
bonding, 1, 29, 35, 52, 104, 114–15, 131
boundaries, 109, 112, 271
Brazil, 9, 11, 16, 35–36, 136
breastfeeding
  difficulties in, 104
  environment and, 89
  hormones and, 113, 114, 115
  nourishment during, 29, 54
  ovulation during, 195
  perfectionism in, 296–97
  sexuality and, 271, 272, 275
  weight loss and, 128
  See also milk production
breath
  awareness of, 71
  full-range, 79
  for length, 72–73, 97, 146, 187, 188,
    253–54
  movement and, 154
  synchronized, 232–33

care providers, assembling network of, 55,
  63, 299–300
cervix, 89, 108, 109, 145, 223, 254, 255, 273
cesarean birth, 16, 69, 103, 223
  body after, 145, 150
  and motherbaby, effect on, 103, 105–6
  recovery from, 146, 170–71
  scar tissue from, 183
  statistics on, 219
  See also VBAC
chakras. See energy centers
chi (life force), 122, 124, 125, 132, 138
childbirth education, 3
Chinese medicine, 140
  belly wrapping in, 149, 150
  benefits of, 142
  energetic body in, 104
  energy channels in, 190–91
  eyes, resting in, 132, 143
  fluids of, 122–24

episiotomy, 176, 183
erotic theme, identifying core, 94–96, 98
Essential Prescriptions (Sun Simiao), 121
Estés, Clarissa Pinkola, 299
estrogen, 111, 113, 180, 271–72
exercise balls, 71, 73, 79, 154, 155, 157

family, 121
  bonding with, 35
  and childbirth, role in, 11, 15
  life, transition to, 3–4, 33, 242, 243,
    277, 299–300
  nuclear model, 198, 293
  partnership relationship in, 229
  Sun Simiao's view of, 121
  support from, 54, 57, 133, 294–95, 299
  in traditional cultures, 152, 204
Family and Medical Leave Act (FMLA), 26
fascia, 181–82
Feldenkrais, 106, 168, 210, 251
feminine, immersion into, 9, 45–46, 47
feminism, 43–44, 304
fetal ejection reflex, 8
fight-or-flight response, 83–84, 89, 115
fire, digestive (agni), 130–31
First Forty Days, The (cookbook), 125
flexibility, 153, 178–79, 251
food, nourishing, 21, 29–31, 99–100, 179
  assembling resources for, 63
  in Chinese medicine, 124–25
  cooking postpartum, 133
  in East and West, differences in, 127
  healthy fats, 139, 179
  help with, 53–54
  meat as, 127
  prioritizing, 119–20, 142
forcep birth, 176, 183, 193
fourth trimester
  celebrating end of, 243
  interconnectedness of mother and baby
    in, 102
  length of, 24–25, 27–28
  opportunities of, 304
  preparing for, 4, 5–6
  rewards of, 99–100
  use of term, 2
  See also postpartum period
freeze response, 87, 89

Freudian analysis, 284
Functional Integration (Feldenkrais), 251.
  See also Feldenkrais

Garza, Keli, 138
Gaskin, Ina May, 89
gender gap, 43–44
gender roles, 228
genitals, 258–59, 260–61
Goddess archetypes, 264
golden hour, 104
golden month, 27, 29
Gottman, John and Julie, 56, 58, 228–29, 239
gratitude, 47, 224, 240, 249–50, 288, 297
grief, 14, 198, 206, 214, 222–23, 224,
  236, 261, 290
grocery list, making sample, 54
Guatemala, 29, 31
Gutman, Laura, 102, 228, 279

Hakomi, 275
Hashimoto's disease, 116
healing
  author's call to help others, 15–18
  author's experience of, 14–15, 184–85,
    196–99
  birth trauma, 217–18
  body as key to, 177
  energy needed for, 49
  factors in, 11
  hands-on, 16
  length of time for, 29
  sex for, 90, 263–64
  trauma, 85
health
  ideals of, 119
  and mothers, relationship to, 292, 300
  postpartum effect on overall, 24, 32,
    121, 304
  radiant, 2, 24, 123, 190, 199
  of women, as central to healthy society,
    121
Heed, Ellen, 13–14, 178, 197, 198
help and support
  asking for, 46, 47, 52
  assembling resources for, 55, 63, 299–300
  planning for, 49–50
  purpose of, 50

hemorrhoids, 11, 13, 14, 175, 258, 259
herbs, 15, 31–32
    Ayurvedic, 131, 132
    in baths, 128, 136
    Chinese, 125, 127
    in teas, 143
    warming, 143
hernias, 188
Holland, 194
homeostasis, 83
Hong Kong, 15, 30
Hopi tradition, 31
hormones, 30, 180
    balancing, 117, 118
    blood work for, 116
    calibration period, 113
    fluctuation, length of time of, 112–13
    hugging and, 233
    immediately after birth, 104, 145
    memory and, 235
    relationships and, 229
    sensitivity from, 51–52
    sex and stress, categories of, 113–14
    sexuality and, 271–72
    stress-related, 37, 83
    support of belly wrapping for, 153
Hulme, Janet, 147
hydration, 137, 140, 142, 179, 182, 183, 274, 318
hypopressives, 253

identity, 199
    evolution of, 246
    feminine, 277
    motherhood and, 5, 25, 43, 204, 227, 279, 290
    in partnerships, shifts in, 241
    reconnecting with, 110
    sexual, 264, 268, 277
    as women, 264
Iemanja, 9
imagination, 256
immune system, 116, 131
impermanence, 249
Inanna, 264
incontinence, 13, 185–86, 200
    author's experience with, 184–85, 191
    fecal, 176, 191

healing, 14
    moxibustion for, 128
    pain in sex from, 275
    posture and, 179
    six-week doctor's visit and, 175
    study on, 69
    tearing and, 189
incorporation phase (rites of passage), 205–6
India, 15, 27, 29, 30, 99, 149, 204
Indo-Malay tradition, 30, 152
infection, minimizing risk of, 125
INNATE Postpartum Care, 204
inner voices/guidance, 41–42, 46, 47, 170
interconnectedness, 293
interdependence, 46, 47, 129, 304
intimacy, 6, 94–96, 97, 241, 242, 259. *See also* sex and sexuality
intuition, 279, 280–81, 285–86, 287, 301
Ionio, Chiara, 211–13

Japan, 27, 136, 204
joints, loosening of, 68
Jordon, Brigitte, 218
joy, 55–56, 250

kapha dosha, 133, 134
Kegel exercises, 77, 78, 97, 153, 186, 254
Kent, Tami Lynn, 118
kindness, 58, 166, 230, 231, 249. *See also* loving-kindness
Korea, 15, 30, 137
Krammzorg maternity care, 194

labia, tearing of, 188–89, 191
labor, 122, 134, 140–42, 168, 176, 206, 209, 210–11
Lang, Raven, 135
laziness, 36, 40
libido, 266
life energy, 131–32, 199
life-force transfer, 25
ligaments, 68–69, 70, 77, 97, 153, 179, 193–94
lotus birth, 102–3
love, 242
    hormones of, 104
    maternal, 288

nervous system, 97
  Ayurvedic view of, 130–31
  baby wearing and, 162
  balancing, 146
  capacity of, 89–90, 93
  cycles of, 83–86
  identifying response of, 88
  massage for settling, 169
  of mother and baby, connection
      between, 101, 104
  training for childbirth, 81–83
  See also parasympathetic nervous
      system; sympathetic nervous system
Northrup, Christiane, 292

Oakes, Ysha, 141, 153
oil, 139–40, 142, 183–84
ojas, revitalizing, 131–32
orgasm, 265
Orgasmic Meditation (OM), 271
osteopathy, 168
overexertion, consequences of, 68, 252–53
ovulation, 195
oxytocin, 114–15, 233

parasympathetic nervous system, 83, 84,
    89, 272
parenting, 300
  communication in, 238–39
  community and, 54–55
  intuition in, 285–86
  relationships and, 56, 58
  revisiting one's own, 227–28
  by single mothers, 294
patience, 249, 250, 257
pelvic diamond, 73
pelvic floor, 97
  baby wearing and, 164
  in belly wrapping, 150
  core and, 147, 148, 149
  damage during childbirth, 8–9, 78, 81
  description of, 74
  dysfunction, emotional factors in, 180–81
  dysfunction, statistics on, 176
  exercise for preparing, 72–73
  finding muscles of, 77–79
  imagery for, 256
  intimacy of, 257

jaw and, 89
  mula bandha for, 254–55
  muscles, 78
  physical therapy for, 79, 81, 98, 147,
      167, 168–69, 175, 197, 251, 275
  tightening of, 68
Pelvic Rotator Cuff (Hulme), 147
pelvic-floor reconstruction, 2, 12, 196–97
pelvis, 167, 168
  health of, four domains, 177–78, 197,
      198, 199, 200, 201
  pain in, 69
  sexuality and, 272
  stabilizing, 77
penetration (PIV), 61
  as cultural norm, 91, 258, 268
  as goal, deconditioning view, 266
  pain during, 274–75
  readiness for, 256, 261, 271–72
  sex without, 93
perfectionism, 43, 47, 296–98, 300
perineum, 80–81, 188–89, 191, 254, 258
physical therapy
  benefits of, 168–69
  for incontinence, 186
  for pelvic floor, 79, 81, 98, 147, 167,
      168–69, 175, 197, 251, 275
  for postpartum period, 6
pitta dosha, 133, 134
placenta, 112, 113, 114, 117, 135
pleasure, 250, 259, 260, 265–66, 274
pornography, 96, 265
postpartum period, 1
  author's experience during, 10–13
  Ayurvedic view of, 130–31
  birth experience and, 66, 225
  creating ritual for, 243
  definitions of, 26–27
  expectations about, 28, 41–43, 47
  fifteen days, first, 146–53
  five universal needs during, 28–32, 51,
      100, 124, 169
  illness in, vulnerability to, 32, 124
  importance of, 142
  as integration rite of passage phase, 206
  posture in, 71
  preparing for, 33–35
  rebuilding strength in, 153–61

reclaiming knowledge about, 3–4
rhythm change in, 41, 47
as time for reevaluation, 247–48
too many "experts" during, 170
vata imbalance in, 134–40
See also fourth trimester
Postpartum Revolution, 5, 23–24, 303–4
posture, *71, 163*
 baby wearing and, *163*–164
 belly wrapping for, 150
 biomechanics of, 178–79
 core rebuilding and, 147
 exercises for, 75
 overhauling, 251
 during pregnancy, 70, *163*
prayer, 106, 132
pregnancy, 65, 69, 122, 145, 204, 206
progesterone, 113, 114, 180
prolapse, 69, *192*
 author's experience with, 184–85
 bandhas for, 253
 causes of, 191–95
 moxibustion for, 128
 pain in sex from, 275
 painful periods after, 195
 posture and, 179
 six-week doctor's visit and, 175
 tearing and, 189
 vaginal steaming for, 138

rasa, 130, 131
rebozo (belly wrapping). *See* belly wrapping
rectus abdominis, 186
relationships, partners and spouses, 63
 balancing personal needs in, 60–61
 birth experience and, 222
 bubble, protecting, 58–59, 231
 checking in, 237–38
 connection and contact in, importance
  of, 231–35
 counseling for, 58
 exercises for maintaining, 230, 232–35,
  237, 238, 240–41
 exploring five love languages in, 61–62
 intimacy building in, 94–96, 97
 limitations of, 49–50
 roles, redefining, 227–28
 safeguarding, 56, 58–60

satisfaction in, 228–29
 staying connected, suggestions for, 62
 unresolved dynamics in, 275
relaxin, 115, 193–94
rest, 99–100
 in Ayurveda, 131, 132
 constructive, 146–47
 extended period of, 28–29
 importance of, 36–37
 learning to, 38, 39–40
 prioritizing, 119–20, 142
 in rebuilding body, 145, 146
rites of passage, 190–91, 225
 birth as, 203
 community and, 207–8
 exercises for, 206–7
 three phases common to, 204–6
Rolf Method of Structural Integration,
 3, 149, 168, 251
running, 252, 261
ruptures and repairs, 295–96

sacred window, 6, 29, 49, 50, 99, 106,
 135, 193, 228
Sacred Window School, 141, 153
sacroiliac joint pain, 69, 77, 147, 150,
 184–85
safety, 87, 89, 104, 108, 209, 272, 295
samskaras, 190–91
sanctuary plan, 35, 49, 50–51, 52, 63
Sankhya philosophy, 129
scar tissue, 181–84
 during delivery, 223
 incontinence and, 186
 pelvic-floor, 197–98
 remediation of, 14
 sexuality and, 259, 271, 272, 274, 275
self-acceptance, 276–77
self-confidence, 66
self-consciousness, biological responses
 and, 84
self-image, 41
self-massage, 139–40
self-regulation, 37, 180
self-sufficiency, ideals of, 57
Seliga, Rachelle Garcia, 204
sensation, expanding capacity for, 93–94
sensitivity, 51–52

uddiyana bandha kriya, 171, 194, 253, 254, 255
ultradian rhythms, 37–38, 39, 40, 47, 83
Unfolding Lap, The (Baker), 245
uterus, 148
    during childbirth, 122, 145, 273
    cleansing of, 29, 125, 137, 138, 195, 260
    prepregnancy size and position, return to, 27, 113, 167, 179, 199
    prolapse of, 191–93
    warmth and, 127, 137

vacuum delivery, 106, 176, 183, 192, 193
vagina, 31, 106, 134, 188–89, 191, 258, 259, 261
vaginal steaming, 136, 137–38, 143, 195, 260
van Gennep, Arnold, 203–6
vata dosha, 132–33, 134, 139, 140, 142, 143, 150
VBAC (vaginal birth after cesarean), 215, 216, 223
vegetarianism, 127, 191, 192, 198
Virgin Mary, 264, 277
visitors, 51–52
Vitti, Alisa, 117
vows, 6, 63
vulvas, 189, 258, 259, 260, 261, 266, 272

walking, 252
warming, 109, 113, 128, 131, 136–37, 142, 150

weight lifting, 261
weight loss, 127, 128
Welch, Claudia, 113
Welm, Sabine, 121
Wild Feminine (Kent), 118
Winnicott, D. W., 295–96, 298
Winston, Sheri, 266
Wired for Love (Tatkin), 58, 231
wolf and rabbit story, 85
WomanCode (Vitti), 117
wombs, honoring, 112, 118
women
    archetypes of, 264, 294
    body image and, 248
    in contemporary society, 23
    discounting experience of, 212
    need for other women of, 293, 294
    rites of passage as built-in, 207
    sexual anatomy of, 265–66
    wise, need for, 30–31, 142, 299
Women Who Run with the Wolves (Estés), 299
Women's Anatomy of Arousal (Winston), 266

yin and yang, 113–14, 122–23, 142
yoga, 4, 109
    bandhas in, 253–55, 261
    energetic body in, 104
    during pregnancy, 67, 69, 77
    for rebuilding strength, 155
yoni eggs, 256

about the author

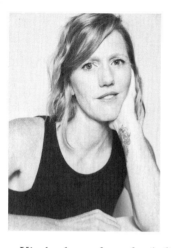

Kimberly Johnson is a birth doula, Sexological Bodyworker, Somatic Experiencing practitioner, postpartum care advocate, and single mom. Kimberly is the cofounder of the STREAM School for Postpartum Care, where she trains birth professionals, bodyworkers, and somatic therapists to help women with prolapse, incontinence, painful sex, and other pelvic-floor and gynecological issues.

Kimberly graduated valedictorian in the School of Education and Social Policy at Northwestern University. A longtime yoga teacher, yoga teacher trainer, and Structural Integration practitioner, she was unexpectedly rearranged in body, mind, and spirit when she sustained an injury during childbirth. Determined not to get full pelvic-floor reconstructive surgery, she traveled the world learning about postpartum practices, healed herself holistically, and now helps other women do the same.

She has private practices in Encinitas and Los Angeles, CA, specializing in helping women prepare for birth, recover from birth injuries and birth trauma, and access their full sexual expression. Her most outstanding accomplishment is being a single mom to her fiery nine-year-old half-Brazilian daughter, Cecilia.

You can find her online at www.magamama.com.